SpringerBriefs in Criminology

SpringerBriefs in Criminology present concise summaries of cutting edge research across the fields of Criminology and Criminal Justice. It publishes small but impactful volumes of between 50-125 pages, with a clearly defined focus. The series covers a broad range of Criminology research from experimental design and methods, to brief reports and regional studies, to policy-related applications.

The scope of the series spans the whole field of Criminology and Criminal Justice, with an aim to be on the leading edge and continue to advance research. The series will be international and cross-disciplinary, including a broad array of topics, including juvenile delinquency, policing, crime prevention, terrorism research, crime and place, quantitative methods, experimental research in criminology, research design and analysis, forensic science, crime prevention, victimology, criminal justice systems, psychology of law, and explanations for criminal behavior.

SpringerBriefs in Criminology will be of interest to a broad range of researchers and practitioners working in Criminology and Criminal Justice Research and in related academic fields such as Sociology, Psychology, Public Health, Economics and Political Science.

More information about this series at http://www.springer.com/series/10159

Wesley G. Jennings • Nicholas Perez
Chris Delcher • Yanning Wang

Opioid Prescribing Rates and Criminal Justice and Health Outcomes

Springer

Wesley G. Jennings
Department of Legal Studies
University of Mississippi
University, MS, USA

Chris Delcher
Department of Pharmacy Practice
and Science
University of Kentucky
Lexington, KY, USA

Nicholas Perez
School of Criminology, Criminal Justice,
and Emergency Management
California State University System
Long Beach, CA, USA

Yanning Wang
Department of Health Outcomes and
Biomedical Informatics
University of Florida
Gainesville, FL, USA

ISSN 2192-8533 ISSN 2192-8541 (electronic)
SpringerBriefs in Criminology
ISBN 978-3-030-40763-6 ISBN 978-3-030-40764-3 (eBook)
https://doi.org/10.1007/978-3-030-40764-3

This Springer imprint is published by the registered company Springer Nature Switzerland AG
The registered company address is: Gewerbestrasse 11, 6330 Cham, Switzerland

Acknowledgments

The authors would like to acknowledge the staff and director of the Controlled Substance Utilization Review and Evaluation System (CURES), Tina Farales, for making California's Prescription Behavior Surveillance System (PBSS) data archive available. In addition, the authors acknowledge the Prescription Drug Monitoring Program (PDMP) Training and Technical Assistance Center (TTAC) at Brandeis University and its efforts to establish and maintain the Prescription Behavior Surveillance System (PBSS) project.

A special thanks to Eugene Shin and Christian Eisinger for creating figures and Nailah Horne for the manuscript review.

This project was supported by Grant No. 2017-PM-BX-K038 awarded by the Bureau of Justice Assistance, which is a component of the Department of Justice's Office of Justice Programs that also includes the Bureau of Justice Statistics, the National Institute of Justice, the Office of Juvenile Justice and Delinquency Prevention, the Office for Victims of Crime, and the SMART Office. Points of view or opinions in this document are those of the authors and do not necessarily represent the official position or policies of the US Department of Justice.

Contents

About the Authors

Wesley G. Jennings, Ph.D. is Chair and Professor in the Department of Legal Studies at the University of Mississippi (Ole Miss). In addition, he also has a Courtesy Appointment in the Department of Health Outcomes and Biomedical Informatics and is a Faculty Affiliate of the Institute for Child Health Policy in the College of Medicine at the University of Florida. He received his doctorate degree in criminology from the University of Florida. He has over 250 publications, his *h*-index is 51 (*i*-index of 152), and he has over 9,000 citations to his published work. He was recognized as the #1 criminologist in the world at his previous rank of Assistant Professor (Copes et al., *JCJE* 2013), the #1 criminologist in the world at his previous rank of Associate Professor (Khey, *JCJE* 2017), and the #3 criminologist in the world *across all ranks* in terms of his peer-reviewed scholarly publication productivity in the top criminology and criminal justice journals (Cohn and Farrington, *JCJE*, 2014). He is the author of several recently published, academic press books with Springer: *Female Delinquency from Childhood to Young Adulthood: Recent Results from the Pittsburgh Girls Study* (with Rolf Loeber, Lia Ahonen, Alex Piquero, and David Farrington); *Offending from Childhood to Young Adulthood: Recent Results from the Pittsburgh Youth Study* (with Rolf Loeber, Dustin Pardini, Alex Piquero, and David Farrington); and *Offending from Childhood to Late Middle Age: Recent Results from the Cambridge Study in Delinquent Development* (with David Farrington and Alex Piquero). In addition, he is the author (with Jennifer Reingle) of the second edition of *Criminological and Criminal Justice Research Methods* (published by Wolters Kluwer) and an author (with Ronald Akers and Christine Sellers) of the seventh edition of *Criminological Theories: Introduction, Evaluation, and Application* (published by Oxford University Press). His major research interests are quantitative methods and longitudinal data analysis. He is a Member of the American Society of Criminology and a Lifetime Member of both the Academy of Criminal Justice Sciences and the Southern Criminal Justice Association. Finally, he is a Fellow of the Academy of Criminal Justice Sciences (ACJS) and is currently the President of the Southern Criminal Justice Association.

Nicholas Perez, Ph.D. is an Assistant Professor in the School of Criminology, Criminal Justice, and Emergency Management at California State University, Long Beach (CSULB). He has authored or coauthored peer-reviewed journal articles in *Aggression and Violent Behavior*, the *Annual Review of Clinical Psychology, Crime & Delinquency*, the *Journal of Contemporary Criminal Justice*, *Policing: An International Journal of Police Strategies and Management*, the *Journal of Youth and Adolescence*, the *Security Journal*, the *Journal of Criminal Justice Education*, and *Child Abuse & Neglect*. His main research interests involve the development of delinquent behavior, policing, and opioid and prescription drug abuse. In addition to his academic appointment, he currently works as a research consultant for a Bureau of Justice Assistance (BJA) grant examining opioid prescription data in California. He is a Member of both the American Society of Criminology and the Western Society of Criminology.

Chris Delcher, Ph.D. is an Epidemiologist and Assistant Professor in the Department of Pharmacy Practice and Science and the Associate Director of the Institute for Pharmaceutical Outcomes and Policy at the University of Kentucky. In addition, he also has a Courtesy Appointment in the Department of Health Outcomes and Biomedical Informatics and is a Faculty Affiliate of the Institute for Child Health Policy in the College of Medicine at the University of Florida. He received his master's degree from the Gillings School of Global Public Health, University of North Carolina, and his Ph.D. in Epidemiology from the University of Florida. He has authored or coauthored more than 50 publications in leading medical and public health journals including the *Annals of Internal Medicine*, the *American Journal of Preventive Medicine*, the *American Journal of Public Health*, *Morbidity and Mortality Weekly Report*, the *Journal of Adolescent Health*, *Drug and Alcohol Dependence*, and *Forensic Science International* and is Coauthor of *Data Driven Approaches for Healthcare: Machine learning for Identifying High Utilizers*. His research focuses on the epidemiology of prescription drug use from data obtained during medical and pharmacy encounters, understanding the intended and unintended consequences of drug policy and its effects on population health, and enhancing public health surveillance systems in high- and low-resource environments.

Yanning Wang, M.S. is a Data Management Analyst in the Department of Health Outcomes and Biomedical Informatics in the College of Medicine at the University of Florida. She has authored or coauthored peer-reviewed journal articles in *JAMA*, the *Annals of Internal Medicine*, the *American Journal of Preventive Medicine*, the *American Journal of Public Health*, *Morbidity and Mortality Weekly Report*, *Drug and Alcohol Dependence*, the *American Journal of Epidemiology*, the *American Journal of Occupational Therapy*, *Accident Analysis & Prevention*, and *Forensic Science International*. Her research focus is injury surveillance and prevention. She currently works on strategic planning for public health initiatives, develops and maintains a drug-related outcomes surveillance system, and leads research on drug abuse and overdose prevention funded by the US Department of Justice, Bureau of Justice Assistance. She was the architect for the first publicly available data-driven surveillance system for monitoring prescription and other drug-related outcomes in Florida. She works closely with public health and public safety agencies to develop prevention strategies to address the ongoing drug overdose epidemic. She has also conducted a series of studies to investigate emerging drug epidemics and evaluate the impact of national drug policies on populations vulnerable to substance abuse.

Chapter 1
Introduction to the Opioid Crisis

The awareness of an opioid epidemic in recent years in the U.S. is nearly ubiquitous, and in 2017, the opioid prescribing rate in the U.S. has been reported to be as high as 17% of Americans having had at least one opioid prescription filled (Robert Wood Johnson Foundation & Harvard T.H. Chan School of Public Health 2018; U.S. Centers for Disease Control and Prevention 2017a, b). Additional evidence has suggested that the opioid dose delivered to recipients in terms of morphine milligram equivalents (MMEs) has tripled from 1999 to 2015, and the average number of days per opioid prescription has increased as well (up from approximately 13 days in 2006 to approximately 18 days in 2017) (U.S. Centers for Disease Control and Prevention 2017b). In 2017, the U.S. Department of Health and Human Services declared a public health emergency to address the opioid crisis and its effects, including misuse, addiction, overdose, and death with multiple states following suit.

While California has not declared a state emergency to address the opioid crisis, the state has developed a comprehensive state-wide approach to address the opioid epidemic with nine strategies and activities: (1) develop a state-wide opioid safety workgroup, (2) promote safe prescribing, (3) build community capacity engagement, (4) expand medication assisted treatment (MAT), (5) increase access to naloxone, (6) reduce access to and negative consequences of illicit drugs, (7) address priority populations in high risk settings, (8) promote public education and awareness, and (9) translate data into actionable information (California Department of Public Health 2018a). The current project aims to meet the final objective by translating California opioid data into more actionable information.

According to the California Department of Public Health (2018b), there were 21,787,042 opioid prescriptions written in California in 2017. Compared to the national average, California has a lower overall opioid prescribing rate. In 2013, California providers wrote approximately 549 opioid prescriptions per 1000 people, while the U.S. rate was 793 per 1000 people (National Institute on Drug Abuse

W. G. Jennings et al., *Opioid Prescribing Rates and Criminal Justice and Health Outcomes*, SpringerBriefs in Criminology,
https://doi.org/10.1007/978-3-030-40764-3_1

2018). Additionally, opioid-related overdose deaths are lower in California (4.9 per 100,000 people) than the nationwide average of 13.3 per 100,000 (National Institute on Drug Abuse 2018) a consistent trend historically.

The adverse public health-related outcomes associated with opioid prescribing behavior in general including increased emergency department use, hospitalization, and overdoses all of which have been well documented in the literature (Baumblatt et al. 2014; Braden et al. 2010; Dilokthornsakul et al. 2016; Ekstrom et al. 2014; Hall et al. 2008; Park et al. 2015). Other studies have examined the nature and extent of high-risk opioid prescribing behavior (Liu et al. 2013; Logan et al. 2013; Mack et al. 2015; Meara et al. 2016; Paulozzi et al. 2015). In general, though, localized opioid prescribing patterns have not yet been sufficiently researched. In recent years, though, a variety of online data systems have increased opioid-related data availability, facilitating research into local opioid prescribing trends, as well as the associates and adverse public health outcomes of them (U.S. Centers for Disease Control 2019). For example, Quast et al. (2018) used data from the Florida Drug-Related Outcomes and Surveillance System to examine the county-level association between opioid prescribing and children removed from the home in Florida.

To address the opioid crisis in the United States, all 50 states have developed some type of Prescription Drug Monitoring Program (PDMP). In California, the PDMP is known as the Controlled Substance Utilization Review and Evaluation System (CURES 2.0). Administered by the California Department of Justice, CURES 2.0 maintains a database of controlled substance prescriptions for public health and law enforcement agencies in efforts to reduce the abuse of prescription drugs, including opioids. In CURES 2.0, all prescribers that are licensed to prescribe schedule II, III, and IV substances were required to register by July 1, 2016 (California Department of Justice 2018). This included all licensed dentists, physicians, nurses, and veterinarians. Additionally, pharmacies, clinics, and other dispensers of these controlled substances were required to provide weekly prescription information to monitor prescribing behaviors (including patient, pharmacy, drug, and prescription information).

The CURES 2.0 system is programmed to monitor when a patient's opioid prescription level exceeds certain thresholds, and beginning in October of 2018, prescribers were required to consult the CURES 2.0 system prior to the first time of prescribing, ordering, or administering a schedule II, III, or IV substance and after every four months of prescribing the drug to a patient (California Department of Justice 2018). In addition to its utility for monitoring abnormal prescribing behavior, the CURES 2.0 data was previously sent to a national Prescription Behavior Surveillance System (PBSS) that compiled prescription data from participating states. The PBSS was conceived as an early warning surveillance system to prevent opioid and other prescription drug abuse and promote safer prescribing practices.

Using the county-level opioid prescribing data collected by the PBSS, the Chapters that follow will present original research on county-level opioid prescribing rates in California from 2012 to 2017 in several phases. Chapter 2 will summarize the general trends in prescribing from 2012 to 2017, comparing opioid prescribing behavior to other controlled substance prescription drugs, and examine specific trends by sex, age, and drug type. Other data related to daily dosage, overlapping days in treatment, multiple provider episodes, opioid-naïve prescribing, and the top opioid prescribers will also be discussed.

For these specific measures, mean daily dosage is calculated for subjects that have a prescription in a quarter and the morphine milligram equivalents prescribed per day (PDMP Training and Technical Assistance Center 2019). Overlapping days in treatment is calculated by the number of days with more than one prescription in the same class of drugs divided by the total prescription days for that class (PDMP Training and Technical Assistance Center 2019). Multiple provider episodes refers to "the use of 5 or more prescribers and 5 or more pharmacies within 3 months and is based on the current 3 months" and is reported each quarter (PDMP Training and Technical Assistance Center 2019). Opioid-naïve prescribing is prescribing to patients with no opioid prescriptions in the previous 60 days (PDMP Training and Technical Assistance Center 2019). Finally, a top opioid prescriber refers to those in the top 1% of opioid prescribing (PDMP Training and Technical Assistance Center 2019).

The three chapters that follow will address the three central research questions related to this book by examining important contextual correlations with California's county-level prescribing rates. Chapter 3 will explore the association of community characteristics in multiple domains (demographics, population density, housing, income, employment, and health) on the opioid prescribing rate. Then, Chap. 4 will assess the association of the opioid prescribing rate on county-level arrest rates (violent, property, drug, and total crimes) in California, while controlling for the other relevant county-level characteristics. Chapter 5 will explore the association of California's county-level opioid prescribing rates on three county-level opioid-related public health outcome rates: emergency room visits, hospitalizations, and fatal overdose deaths, while controlling for the other relevant county-level characteristics. Finally, Chap. 6 will summarize the main findings of this project, highlighting the policy implications of the results, and discussing future directions for opioid prescribing practices and criminal justice and public health outcomes.

References

Baumblatt, J. A. G., Wiedeman, C., Dunn, J. R., Schaffner, W., Paulozzi, L. J., & Jones, T. F. (2014). High-risk use by patients prescribed opioids for pain and its role in overdose deaths. *JAMA Internal Medicine, 174*(5), 796–801.

Braden, J. B., Russo, J., Fan, M.-Y., Edlund, M. J., Martin, B. C., DeVries, A., & Sullivan, M. D. (2010). Emergency department visits among recipients of chronic opioid therapy. *Archives of Internal Medicine, 170*(16), 1425–1432.

California Department of Justice (2018). *Controlled substance utilization review and evaluation system.* Retrieved from https://oag.ca.gov/cures.

California Department of Public Health (2018a). *California's approach to the opioid epidemic.* Retrieved from https://www.cdph.ca.gov/Pages/Opioids.aspx

California Department of Public Health (2018b). *California opioid overdose surveillance dashboard.* Retrieved from https://discovery.cdph.ca.gov/CDIC/ODdash/

Dilokthornsakul, P., Moore, G., Campbell, J. D., Lodge, R., Traugott, C., Zerzan, J., et al. (2016). Risk factors of prescription opioid overdose among Colorado Medicaid beneficiaries. *The Journal of Pain, 17*(4), 436–443.

Ekstrom, M. P., Bornefalk-Hermansson, A., Abernethy, A. P., & Currow, D. C. (2014). Safety of benzodiazepines and opioids in very severe respiratory disease: National prospective study. *BMJ (Clinical Research Ed.), 348*, g445.

Hall, A. J., Logan, J. E., Toblin, R. L., Kaplan, J. A., Kraner, J. C., Bixler, D., et al. (2008). Patterns of abuse among unintentional pharmaceutical overdose fatalities. *Journal of the American Medical Association, 300*(22), 2613–2620.

Liu, Y., Logan, J. E., Paulozzi, L. J., Zhang, K., & Jones, C. M. (2013). Potential misuse and inappropriate prescription practices involving opioid analgesics. *The American Journal of Managed Care, 19*(8), 648–665.

Logan, J., Liu, Y., Paulozzi, L., Zhang, K., & Jones, C. (2013). Opioid prescribing in emergency departments: The prevalence of potentially inappropriate prescribing and misuse. *Medical Care, 51*(8), 646–653.

Mack, K. A., Zhang, K., Paulozzi, L., & Jones, C. (2015). Prescription practices involving opioid analgesics among Americans with Medicaid, 2010. *Journal of Health Care for the Poor and Underserved, 26*(1), 182–198.

Meara, E., Horwitz, J. R., Powell, W., McClelland, L., Zhou, W., O'Malley, A. J., & Morden, N. E. (2016). State legal restrictions and prescription-opioid use among disabled adults. *New England Journal of Medicine, 375*(1), 44–53.

National Institute on Drug Abuse (2018). *California opioid summary*. Retrieved from https://www.drugabuse.gov/drugs-abuse/opioids/opioid-summaries-by-state/california-opioid-summary.

Park, T. W., Saitz, R., Ganoczy, D., Ilgen, M. A., & Bohnert, A. S. B. (2015). Benzodiazepine prescribing patterns and deaths from drug overdose among U.S. veterans receiving opioid analgesics: Case-cohort study. *BMJ (Clinical Research Ed.), 350*, h2698.

Paulozzi, L. J., Strickler, G. K., Kreiner, P. W., & Koris, C. M. (2015). Controlled substance prescribing patterns—prescription behavior surveillance system, eight states, 2013. *MMWR Surveillance Summaries, 64*(9), 1–14.

PDMP Training and Technical Assistance Center (2019). *Prescription behavior surveillance system*. Retrieved from https://www.pdmpassist.org/content/prescription-behavior-surveillance-system

Quast, T., Storch, E. A., & Yampolskaya, S. (2018). Opioid prescription rates and child removals: Evidence from Florida. *Health Aff (Millwood), 37*(1), 134–139.

Robert Wood Johnson Foundation & Harvard T.H. Chan School of Public Health (2018). Life in rural America. NPR. Retrieved from https://www.rwjf.org/en/library/research/2018/10/life-in-rural-america.html

U.S. Centers for Disease Control (2019). *Opioid data analysis and resources*. Retrieved from https://www.cdc.gov/drugoverdose/data/analysis.html

U.S. Centers for Disease Control and Prevention (2017a). *Prescription opioid data*. U.S. Department of Health and Human Services. Retrieved from https://www.cdc.gov/drugoverdose/data/prescribing.html.

U.S. Centers for Disease Control and Prevention (2017b). *2018 Annual surveillance report of drug-related risks and outcomes*. U.S. Department of Health and Human Services. Retrieved from. https://www.cdc.gov/drugoverdose/pdf/pubs/2018-cdc-drug-surveillance-report.pdf.

Chapter 2
County-Level Prescribing Rates: Aggregated and Disaggregated

2.1 California's Prescription Behavior Surveillance System (PBSS)

Data on the prescribing rates for each county in California was obtained through the PBSS, which is a system that allows public health entities to measure the use and misuse of various prescription controlled substances, including opioids. The PBSS was funded by the U.S. Centers for Disease Control (CDC) and the Food and Drug Administration (FDA) and hosted by the Bureau of Justice Assistance (BJA) in contract with Brandeis University's Prescription Drug Monitoring Program (PDMP) Center of Excellence (PDMP Training and Technical Assistance Center 2019). In this system, participating state PDMPs collect and submit prescription data to the PBSS to facilitate comparisons in the rates of prescription drugs based on various other measures, such as demographics, drug types, and daily dose. California's county-level prescription data was collected quarterly since 2012. The analyses in this book focus on the California PBSS data from 2012 to 2017 (most recent data available) (see Appendix 1 for visual illustrations to accompany the descriptive data presented in this chapter).

2.2 Aggregated County-Level Prescribing Rates

Opioids are classified in the PBSS as a class of drugs used to treat moderate to severe pain using the therapeutic code from the Red Book (U.S. Centers for Disease Control 2019). Opioids included: Buprenorphine, Butraphanol, Codeine, Dihydrocodeine, Fentanyl LA, Fentanyl SA, Hydrocodone LA, Hydrocodone SA, Hydromorphone, Meperidine, Methadone, Morphine LA, Morphine SA, Oxycodone

W. G. Jennings et al., *Opioid Prescribing Rates and Criminal Justice and Health Outcomes*, SpringerBriefs in Criminology,
https://doi.org/10.1007/978-3-030-40764-3_2

LA, Oxycodone SA, Oxymorphone LA, Oxymorphone SA, Pentazocine, Tapentadol, Tramadol LA [beginning in August 2014], Tramadol SA [beginning in August 2014], and an "other" category. On average, opioid prescribing has decreased in California from 2012 to 2017. Overall, the data suggests that most counties have experienced a decline in their opioid prescribing rates during this study period. Specifically, from 2012 to 2017, 52 of the 58 counties in California experienced a decline in their annual opioid prescribing rate. Only Alpine, Fresno, Imperial, Kern, Riverside, and San Bernardino observed an increase in their average quarterly opioid prescribing rate from 2012 to 2017. Overall, the average quarterly opioid prescribing rate in 2012 was 232.28 per 1000 residents and ranged from a low of 46.97 per 1000 residents to a high of 453.59 per 1000 residents. In 2017, the average quarterly prescribing rate was 197.97 per 1000 residents and ranged from a low of 84.04 per 1000 residents to a high of 337.38 per 1000 residents.

Stimulants are classified in the PBSS as a class of drugs used to increase alertness, attention, and energy (U.S. Centers for Disease Control 2019). Stimulants included: Amphetamine, Benzphetamine, Dexmethylphenidate, Dextroamphetamine, Lisdexamfetamine, Methylphenidate, and an "other" category. On average, stimulant prescribing has increased in California from 2012 to 2017. Contrary to the opioid trends, the data suggests that most counties have experienced an increase in their stimulant prescribing rates from 2012 to 2017. Specifically, all but seven counties in California experienced an increase in their annual stimulant prescription rate. Only Lassen, Mariposa, Nevada, Plumas, Sierra, Tulare, and Tuolumne observed a decrease in their annual prescribing rate of stimulants from 2012 to 2017. Overall, the average stimulant prescribing rate in 2012 was 23.38 per 1000 residents and ranged from a low of 6.75 per 1000 residents to a high of 37 per 1000 residents. In 2017, the average annual prescribing rate had increased to 28.73 per 1000 residents.

Benzodiazepines are classified in the PBSS as a class of sedative drugs used to treat anxiety, insomnia, and other conditions (U.S. Centers for Disease Control 2019). Benzodiazepines included: Alprazolam, Chlordiazepoxide, Clonazepam, Clorazepate, Diazepam, Estazolam, Flurazepam, Lorazepam, Oxazepam, Temazepam, Triazolam, and an "other" category). Benzodiazepine prescribing has decreased in California from 2012 to 2017. Though substantially lower, the benzodiazepine trends more closely resemble opioid prescribing trends during this time period likely due to the high rates of co-prescribing with opioids. In fact, 56 of the 58 counties in California experienced a decline in their annual benzodiazepine prescribing rate. Only Alpine and Fresno observed an increase in their annual benzodiazepine prescribing rate from 2012 to 2017. Overall, the average annual benzodiazepine prescribing rate in 2012 was 103.63 per 1000 residents and ranged from a low of 25 per 1000 residents to a high of 189.75. In 2017, the average annual prescribing rate was 85.55 per 1000 residents with a low of 28.05 per 1000 residents to a high of 133.2 per 1000 residents.

2.3 County-Level Prescribing Rates by Sex

Concerning opioids, on average, in 2012, females had higher prescribing rates (per 1000 residents) than males (262.75 vs. 202.29). This difference persisted in relative terms but both rates were decreased in 2017 (222.34 for females compared to 173.65 for males). In 2012, opioid prescribing rates for females exceeded the male rates in nearly all of the counties in California with the exception of Alpine, Lassen, Mono, and San Francisco. In 2017, however, male prescribing rates surpassed females in 20 of the 58 counties due to higher prescribing for males and lower prescribing for females over the study period. Regarding stimulants, on average, in 2012, females had higher prescribing rates (per 1000 residents) than males (24.41 vs. 22.27). While the average quarterly rates did change over time, this relative difference in stimulant prescriptions for females and males remained each year. Overall, both rates had increased in 2017 to 31.33 for females and up to 26.29 for males. Finally, on average, in 2012, females had significantly higher benzodiazepine prescribing rates (per 1000 residents) than males (134.41 vs. 72.5). Similar to opioid prescribing rates, the benzodiazepine prescribing rates decreased over time, reaching a study-period low in 2017 of 109.17 for females and 61.72 for males.

2.4 County-Level Prescribing Rates by Age

The data largely reflects that in 2012 (12.22 per 1000 residents) and 2017 (10.24 per 1000 residents), individuals under the age of 18 had the lowest rate of opioid prescriptions and only increased slightly for the 18–24 age group. Depending on the county, the highest rates of opioid prescriptions were found for those in older age groups, such as 45–54, 55–64 and over the age of 65. Comparatively, on average, stimulant prescribing rates generally decreased with age. In 2012, individuals under the age of 18 had the highest rate of simulant prescriptions (34.57 per 1000 residents), but in 2017, individuals in the age range of 35–44 had the highest rate (38.12 per 1000 residents). The lowest rate of stimulant prescriptions was found for those age 65 and up in both 2012 (8.1 per 1000 residents) and 2017 (12.03 per 1000 residents). Finally, in the majority of counties, benzodiazepine prescribing rates increased in higher age groups. For example, in 2012 (3.91 per 1000 residents) and 2017 (4.38 per 1000 residents), individuals under the age of 18 had the lowest rate of benzodiazepine prescriptions. In 2012 and 2017, the highest benzodiazepine rate was found for the group over the age of 65 (192.66 and 177.91, respectively). It should be noted that this age trend in benzodiazepine prescribing these counties in 2012 and 2017 is quite similar to the opioid prescribing trends reported earlier in this chapter.

2.5 County-Level Prescribing Rates by Major Types of Drugs

Hydrocodone SA was found to be the most commonly prescribed opioid in all counties. Comparing 2017 to 2012, the majority of counties reported lower rates for Codeine (45 out of 58 counties), Fentanyl LA (55 out of 58 counties), Methadone (57 of 58 counties), and Morphine LA (42 of 58 counties). Oxycodone SA, on the other hand, was prescribed at a higher rate in 2017 in all but 12 counties in California.

The most commonly prescribed of the two stimulants varied by county and year. On average, though, Amphetamine was prescribed at a higher rate than Methylphenidate in 2012 (7.21 compared to 5.71 per 1000 residents) and 2017 (9.79 compared to 6.36 per 1000 residents). Comparing 2017 to 2012, the majority of counties reported higher rates for Amphetamine (54 out of 58 counties) in 2017, but only half of all counties reported higher prescribing rates of Methylphenidate (29 out of 58 counties) in 2017.

On average, in 2012, Lorazepam was found to be the most commonly prescribed benzodiazepine in California (30.1 per 1000 residents), only slightly ahead of Alprazolam (28.64 per 1000 residents). On average, in 2017, all five benzodiazepines had lower prescribing rates than reported in 2012. In fact, the vast majority of counties reported lower prescribing rates for all five substances in 2017: Alprazolam (53 out of 58 counties), Clonazepam (46 out of 58 counties), Diazepam (57 of 58 counties), Lorazepam (52 of 58 counties), and Temazepam (53 of 58 counties).

On average, Zolpidem was prescribed at a higher rate than Carisoprodol in 2012 (36.36 compared to 14.24 per 1000 residents) and in 2017 (23.43 compared to 5.9 per 1000 residents). The vast majority of counties reported lower rates for both Carisoprodol (56 out of 58 counties) in 2017 and all 58 counties reported lower rates of Zolpidem in 2017 than in 2012.

2.6 County-Level Prescribing Rates by Mean Daily Dosage

In both 2012 and 2017, Fentanyl LA had the highest mean daily dosage (MME = 211.98 in 2012 and MME = 182.16 in 2017) of the six most commonly prescribed opioids. In general, the MME was reduced in all six of the most prescribed opioids from 2012 to 2017.

2.7 County-Level Prescribing Rates by Days in Treatment

The average percentage of overlapping days in 2012 by county (averaged by quarter) was 15.29%. The average percentage of overlapping days in treatment increased to 15.43% in 2013, but then decreased each year in 2014 (15.36%), 2015 (14.30%), 2016 (14.10%), and 2017 (12.97%). This is a relatively positive trend given the overdose risks associated with overlapping prescriptions of opioids and benzodiazepines (U.S. Centers for Disease Control 2019).

2.8 County-Level Prescribing Rates by Multiple Provider Episode Rates

The average rate of multiple provider episodes (per 100,000 residents) for opioids in 2012 by county was 8.79. This rate declined each year, falling to 7.64 in 2013, 7.4 in 2014, 5.31 in 2015, 3.13 in 2016, and 2.41 in 2017.

Compared to opioids, the rate of multiple provider episodes was much lower for stimulants. The average rate of multiple provider episodes (per 100,000 residents) for stimulants in 2012 by county was 0.81. This rate fluctuated over time, staying at 0.81 in 2013, decreasing in 2014 (0.73), 2015 (0.59), and 2016 (0.31), before increasing again slightly to 0.38 in 2017.

The average rate of multiple provider episodes for benzodiazepines was higher than stimulants, but still did not reach the levels of opioids each year. The average rate of multiple provider episodes (per 100,000 residents) for stimulants in 2012 by county was 5.77. Similar to the trend in opioid multiple provider episodes, this rate declined each year, falling to 5.15 in 2013, 5.05 in 2014, 3.56 in 2015, 2.12 in 2016, and 1.48 in 2017.

2.9 County-Level Prescribing Rates for Opioid Naïve Patients

In 2012, the average percentage of LA/ER opioids prescribed to opioid naïve patients was 16.98%. This percentage of prescriptions fluctuated each year, reaching its peak at 36.13% in 2015, but ultimately dropped to 14.91% in 2017.

The average daily dosage for opioid naïve patients changed slightly each year, but overall, did not have any major variations. In 2012, the average annual daily dosage was 168.8 MMEs. In 2013, it increased slightly to 170.84, only to fall to 153.53 in 2014. Over the next three years, the rate rose to 170.05 (2015), fell slightly to 167.12 (2016), and then reached a study-period high of 176.16 MMEs in 2017.

2.10 County-Level Prescribing Rates by Top 1% of Prescribers

Past research has indicated that the top 1% of prescribers are more likely to be sanctioned for inappropriate prescribing and their overprescribing is linked to opioid-related overdoses (Kreiner et al. 2017). While counties reported distinct averages each quarter, of the 50 counties included, the mean number of opioid prescriptions written per day was 12.25. This number fluctuated very slightly over time (12.36 in 2013, 12.3 in 2014, 12.87 in 2015, 12.68 in 2016, 12.2 in 2017), but very little change was found each year. On average, the top 1% of opioid prescribers reported a relatively stable prescribing rate from 2012 to 2017.

The percentage of opioid prescriptions written by the top 1% of prescribers increased somewhat over time from 13.5% in 2012 to 15.57% in 2017. As a note, this annual average excludes counties with 0% written by the top 1% of prescribers. If all counties are included, the percentage increased from 11.6% in 2012 to 13.4% in 2017. On average, the top 1% of opioid prescribers made up a larger percentage of opioid prescriptions in 2017 than in 2012.

2.11 Summary

The current chapter summarized the quarterly county-level PBSS data on opioid, stimulant, and benzodiazepine prescribing rates in California for 2012 to 2017. To compare the opioid prescribing rates to other prescriptions, this data was presented at the aggregate level, and separated by sex and age. Furthermore, the data was summarized for the most commonly prescribed opioids, stimulants, benzodiazepines, and other miscellaneous controlled substance prescription drugs. Finally, this chapter reported on opioid trends in mean daily dosage for common opioids, overlapping days in treatment with benzodiazepines, multiple provider episodes for opioids, stimulants, benzodiazepines, opioid-naïve patient prescribing, and the top 1% of opioid prescribers. The latter measures are generally thought to be associated with high-risk prescribing behaviors.

Primarily, from 2012 to 2017, opioids were prescribed at a higher rate than stimulants and benzodiazepines. Although most counties experienced a decline in opioid prescribing, it remains substantially higher than the other prescribing rates. Furthermore, these reductions in opioid prescribing are not universal at the county-level. Generally, prescribing rates for females exceeded that for males in all three prescription types. As it pertains to opioids, both male and female rates declined, but this decrease was more widespread for females than males.

Opioids were more often prescribed to older patients. This trend was also generally found for benzodiazepines, but not for stimulants, where younger patients received higher prescription rates. When examining six of the most commonly prescribed opioids, Hydrocodone SA was most commonly prescribed. All opioid prescribing rates, with the exception of Oxycodone SA, decreased over time. While this finding of increased Oxycodone SA prescribing is descriptive, Barnett et al. (2018) reported that after a large health insurer in California implemented policies to require prior authorization of Oxycodone LA, increasing barriers to prescribing, there was an slight offsetting increase in prescribing of Oxycodone SA. In general, the mean daily doses for all six of the most commonly prescribed opioids also declined from 2012 to 2017.

From 2012 to 2017, the overlapping days of treatment for opioids and benzodiazepines decreased. Multiple provider episode rates for opioids also declined from 2012 to 2017. Despite having much lower rates than opioids, benzodiazepine multiple provider episodes also declined, while stimulants fluctuated without any clear pattern. Comparing 2017 to 2012, opioid naïve patients were found to receive a smaller proportion of the overall prescriptions, but the mean daily dosage was slightly higher. Finally, despite writing about the same number of prescriptions, the top 1% of opioid prescribers wrote a larger percentage of opioid prescriptions in 2017 than in 2012.

This research has presented a preliminary step in summarizing data on opioid prescribing rates at the county-level and comparing it to other controlled substance prescription rates. However, this chapter only summarized the data collected by the PBSS and did not provide any context on potential correlates of these trends or the consequences of them. The forthcoming chapters (Chaps. 3, 4, and 5) will address these issues by answering three key research questions using this 2012 to 2017 opioid prescribing data: (1) What are the associations between community characteristics (demographics, population density, housing, income, employment, and health) and the opioid prescribing rate? (2) What are the associations between the opioid prescribing rate and county-level arrest rates? and (3) What are the associations between the opioid prescribing rate and county-level opioid-related public health outcome rates? These analyses will assist in further contextualizing opioid prescribing practices in California.

References

Barnett, M. L., Olenski, A. R., Thygeson, N. M., et al. (2018). A health plan's formulary led to reduced use of extended-release opioids but did not lower overall opioid use. *Health Affairs, 37*(9), 1509–1516.

Kreiner, P. W., Strickler, G. K., Undurraga, E. A., Torres, M. E., Nikitin, R. V., & Rogers, A. (2017). Validation of prescriber risk indicators obtained from prescription drug monitoring program data. *Drug and Alcohol Dependence, 173*, S31–S38.

PDMP Training and Technical Assistance Center (2019). *Prescription behavior surveillance system*. Retrieved from https://www.pdmpassist.org/content/prescription-behavior-surveillance-system

U.S. Centers for Disease Control (2019) *Opioid data analysis and resources*. Retrieved from https://www.cdc.gov/drugoverdose/data/analysis.html

Chapter 3
Association Between Community Characteristics and Opioid Prescribing Rates

Several studies have identified individual-level factors such as patient gender (female), race (White) and age (older) (Hwang et al. 2016; Liu et al. 2013; Paulozzi et al. 2015; Yang et al. 2015) as being significantly associated with higher opioid prescribing behaviors. For example, recent research has estimated that females represent nearly 60% of opioid recipients (Hwang et al. 2016; Liu et al. 2013). Compared to males, females also reported higher rates of past-year (5.9%–4.2%) and lifetime (15.9%–11.2%) use (Back et al. 2010). In addition, for equivalent levels of pain, White patients are significantly more likely to be prescribed opioids than patients of other races (Joynt et al. 2013; Pletcher et al. 2008). Furthermore, prescription rates reportedly peak in the 45–54 and 55–64 age groups (Paulozzi et al. 2015) with nearly one-third of all opioid prescriptions being prescribed to patients in these age ranges (Hwang et al. 2016). These findings are also consistent with the California data summarized in Chap. 2 of this book.

Population-level research focused on county-level measures has reported certain contextual characteristics including demographics, rurality, poverty, unemployment, disabled population, and community disadvantage as being significantly associated with opioid prescribing behavior (Guy et al. 2017; Heins et al. 2018; Stein et al. 2015). For example, in a study of retail prescription data, county-level patterns revealed that counties in the highest quartile of opioid prescriptions had distinguishing characteristics (Guy et al. 2017). Specifically, the counties in the highest quartile had a larger percentage of: White residents, residents living in a micropolitan/rural area, residents over the age of 35, residents without a high school diploma, unemployment, and residents living below the poverty line (Guy et al. 2017). These findings provide preliminary evidence suggesting differential prescribing behaviors across counties in the U.S. and highlight the possibility that certain structural factors may be related to this variation in opioid prescribing behavior.

As of current date, all U.S. states have developed and implemented some form of a PDMP in an effort to address the opioid crisis. In California, the PDMP system/

W. G. Jennings et al., *Opioid Prescribing Rates and Criminal Justice and Health Outcomes*, SpringerBriefs in Criminology,
https://doi.org/10.1007/978-3-030-40764-3_3

program is referred to as the Controlled Substance Utilization Review and Evaluation System (CURES 2.0), and all licensed prescribers of Schedule II, III, and IV substances are required to register with CURES 2.0 (as of July 1, 2016) (California Department of Justice 2018). Relevant to the current chapter, the data that is collected in the CURES 2.0 system is also sent to the national PBSS, which is a database that serves an early warning system for identifying prescription drug abuse and to encourage safer prescribing practices. Recent evidence indicates that the annual opioid prescribing rate in California is approximately 550 prescriptions per 1000 persons (California Department of Public Health 2018), and an opioid overdose death rate at nearly 5 per 100,000 persons in California (National Institute on Drug Abuse 2018).

3.1 Research Question 1

Prior research has been limited to studies at the individual-level, restricted to a single year in time, fairly narrow in terms of community characteristics examined (when included), and have largely been descriptive. As such, the current chapter seeks to provide an in-depth examination of the association of a series of community characteristics (demographics, population density, housing, income, employment, and health) on 2012–2017 opioid prescribing rate for all 58 counties in the state of California. In addition, the association between these community characteristics and the opioid prescribing rates are examined in a multivariable framework in order to assess the robustness of any association with the opioid prescribing rate, while controlling for other relevant factors.

3.2 Data Sources

Two primary data sources were used for this analysis: (1) U.S. Census Bureau (2017) data; and (2) California PBSS data (described in Chap. 2).

3.3 Dependent Variable

The outcome variable of interest is the opioid prescribing rate (which includes: Butraphanol, Codeine, Dihydrocodeine, Fentanyl LA, Fentanyl SA, Hydrocodone LA, Hydrocodone SA, Hydromorphone, Meperidine, Methadone, Morphine LA, Morphine SA, Oxycodone LA, Oxycodone SA, Oxymorphone LA, Oxymorphone SA, Pentazocine, and Tapentadol) for each county in California from 2012 to 2017. In an effort to ease interpretation and to better permit an examination of the association between macro-level characteristics and opioid prescribing rates in general, we averaged/smoothed the data by adding up the quarterly rates for 2012 and 2017, respectively, and dividing by 24 quarters in order to create a 6-year average rate for each county for 2012–2017 (per 1000 residents).

3.4 Community Characteristics

Measures from the U.S. Census Bureau's American Community Survey (2017) were identified and selected based on their theoretical and/or empirical relevance (Curtis et al. 2006; Guy et al. 2017; Pratt and Cullen 2005; Shaw and McKay 1942). Three measures were included in the demographic domain: percent female, percent White, and percent age 18 or younger. Population characteristics of the county were also included using a measure of population per square mile (rurality). Housing characteristics of the county were examined through a measure of residential stability: the percentage of persons living in the same house as one year ago. The economic conditions were measured as percent poverty and percent unemployed. Finally, health characteristics were measured as percent disabled (related to hearing, vision, cognitive, ambulatory, self-care, and independent living) under the age of 65.

3.5 Analytic Strategy

To assess the associations between these community characteristics and the opioid prescribing rate in California counties from 2012 to 2017, two primary stages of analysis were performed using Stata 15.0. In the first stage of the analysis, descriptive and summary statistics are reported for the opioid prescribing rate and the community characteristics. In the second stage of the analysis, the association between the opioid prescribing rate and the community characteristics is examined in a series of regression models. Due to the fact that the dependent variable was represented as a rate and because of the apparent skewness present in the distribution of the opioid prescribing rate, Poisson regression models were estimated to produce standardized regression coefficients (Osgood 2000). Specifically, a separate Poisson regression model was estimated for each type of community characteristics (demographic, population, housing, income, employment, and health) to assess the independent and direct association of each characteristic on the opioid prescribing rate. In contrast, a final multivariable Poisson regression model was estimated in order to investigate the associations between the characteristics and the opioid prescribing rate in a multivariable framework, i.e., while controlling for the other characteristics.

Table 3.1 California county-level descriptive statistics of demographic, population, housing, income, employment, and health characteristics and 2012–2017 opioid prescribing rates (n = 58)

Variables	M	SD	Minimum	Maximum
Demographic characteristics				
% Female	49.50	2.12	37.50	51.70
% White	81.05	10.62	50.20	93.90
% Age 18 and younger	22.05	4.18	13.40	30.90
Population characteristics				
Population per square mile	663.25	2314.75	1.60	17179.10
Housing characteristics				
%Residential stability	84.97	3.70	73.90	94.90
Income characteristics				
% Poverty	15.13	4.84	6.60	25.50
Employment characteristics				
% Unemployed	14.93	4.12	8.40	27.00
Health characteristics				
% Disabled under age 65	9.69	3.76	3.10	18.60
Opioid prescribing rates				
Opioid prescribing rate (2012–2017)	221.86	80.93	64.12	1416.42

*Rates are per 1000 residents

3.6 Results

Table 3.1 presents the descriptive statistics of each of the community characteristics included in the analysis (n = 58). On average, California counties (n = 58) were 49.50% female (SD = 2.12), 81.05% White (SD = 10.62), and 22.05% were 18 years old or younger (SD = 4.18). The average population per square mile was 663.25 (SD = 2314.75). The average percent of people living in the same house as one year ago was 84.97% (SD = 3.70) and the average percent poverty was 15.13% (SD = 4.84). On average, the counties reported 14.93% unemployment (SD = 4.12) and 9.69% of the population being disabled residents under the age of 65 (SD = 3.76). Finally, the mean county-level annual opioid prescribing rate (averaged quarterly; per 1000 residents) from 2012 to 2017 was 221.86 (SD = 80.93).

Table 3.2 presents the standardized regression estimates of the relationship between community characteristics and 2012–2017 opioid prescribing rates in California.[1] The first six columns report the standardized regression estimates for each community characteristic. Percent White ($\beta = 1.203, p < 0.001$) and percent of population age 18 and younger ($\beta = 0.931, p < 0.001$) were both significantly associated with the county-level opioid prescribing rates from 2012–2017. Specifically, counties with higher percentages of people identifying as White and lower percentages of persons age 18 or younger had higher rates of opioid prescriptions. Higher

[1] Multicollinearity was not a concern for these analysis as all of the Variance Inflation Factors (VIF) were below 2.0 (Allison 1999).

Table 3.2 Standardized regression estimates of the association between California county-level demographic, population, housing, income, employment, and health characteristics and 2012–2017 opioid prescribing rates (n = 58)

Variables	Opioid prescribing rate (2012–2017) Est. (% change)	Opioid prescribing rate (2012–2017) Est. (% change)	Opioid prescribing rate (2012–2017) Est. (% change)	Opioid prescribing rate (2012–2017) Est. (% change)	Opioid prescribing rate (2012–2017) Est. (% change)	Opioid prescribing rate (2012–2017) Est. (% change)	Opioid prescribing rate (2012–2017) Est. (% change)
Demographic characteristics							
% Female	1.001 (+0.1%)						1.099*** (+9.9%)
% White	1.203*** (+20.3%)						1.110*** (+11.0%)
% Age 18 and younger	0.931*** (-6.9%)						0.945*** (-5.5%)
Population characteristics							
Population per square mile		0.835*** (-16.5%)					0.965* (-3.5%)
Housing characteristics							
% Residential stability			0.959*** (-4.1%)				0.975*** (-2.5%)
Income characteristics							
% Poverty				1.125*** (+12.5%)			0.985 (-1.5%)
Employment characteristics							
% Unemployed					1.121*** (+12.1%)		1.028* (+2.8%)

(continued)

Table 3.2 (continued)

Variables	Opioid prescribing rate (2012–2017) Est. (% change)	Opioid prescribing rate (2012–2017) Est. (% change)	Opioid prescribing rate (2012–2017) Est. (% change)	Opioid prescribing rate (2012–2017) Est. (% change)	Opioid prescribing rate (2012–2017) Est. (% change)	Opioid prescribing rate (2012–2017) Est. (% change)	Opioid prescribing rate (2012–2017) Est. (% change)
Health characteristics							
% Disabled under age 65						1.279*** (+27.9%)	1.234*** (+23.4%)
-Log likelihood=	-813.02	-948.85	-1038.83	-961.76	-962.93	-643.36	-1060.03
Pseudo R^2=	0.23	0.10	0.01	0.08	0.08	0.39	0.50

Est. = Estimates; estimates represent standardized Poisson regression coefficients

% Change reflects the percent increase/decrease in the opioid prescribing rate for every standard deviation increase in the independent variable

*$p < .05$

**$p < .01$

***$p < .001$

population density was found to be significantly associated with lower opioid prescribing rates ($\beta = 0.835, p < 0.001$). A higher percentage of residential stability was determined to be significantly associated with a lower county-level opioid prescribing rate ($\beta = 0.959$, $p < 0.001$). A higher percentage of those living in poverty was significantly associated with a higher opioid prescribing rate ($\beta = 1.125, p < 0.001$). Higher unemployment was significantly associated with a higher county-level opioid prescribing rate ($\beta = 0.959, p < 0.001$). Finally, a higher percentage of the population who is disabled under the age of 65 was significantly associated with a higher county-level opioid prescribing rate ($\beta = 1.279, p < 0.001$).

Given the significant relationships detailed above, the final stage of the analysis (illustrated in the seventh column) reports the results from a multivariable Poisson regression model that includes all measures entered into the model simultaneously. In this full model, percent female ($\beta = 1.099$, $p < 0.001$) and percent White ($\beta = 1.110$, $p < 0.001$) were both significantly associated with higher opioid prescribing rates from 2012 to 2017. In other words, each one-unit standard deviation increase in percent female in a county was associated with a 9.9% increase in the opioid prescribing rate, and each one-unit standard deviation increase in percent of people identifying as White in a county was associated with an 11.0% increase in the opioid prescribing rate, controlling for all other community characteristics. The percent of the population age 18 and younger was significantly associated with lower opioid prescribing rates ($\beta = 0.945, p < 0.001$). Additionally, a larger population density ($\beta = 0.965$, $p < 0.05$) and higher residential stability ($\beta = 0.975$, $p < 0.001$) remained significantly associated with lower opioid prescribing rates. Finally, a larger unemployment percentage ($\beta = 1.028$, $p < 0.05$) and a larger percentage of those disabled under the age of 65 ($\beta = 1.234, p < 0.001$) were both significantly associated with higher opioid prescribing rates. This indicates that every one-unit standard deviation increase in the percent unemployed in a county and in the percent disabled under the age of 65 in a county was associated with a 2.8% and a 23.4% increase in the county-level opioid prescribing rate, respectively, controlling for all other community characteristics.

3.7 Summary

The current chapter sought to offer an in-depth investigation of the association between community characteristics and the opioid prescribing rates in California for 2012–2017. A number of key findings emerged from this analysis and are briefly highlighted below.

For example, the findings indicate that each type of community characteristic including demographics, population density, housing, income, employment, and health characteristics were independently and significantly associated with the 2012–2017 opioid prescribing rate. Furthermore, the associations were in the expected direction and consistent with the literature, as counties with a higher percentage of females, people identifying as White, and older persons were associated with higher opioid prescribing rates (Hwang et al. 2016; Liu et al. 2013; Paulozzi et al. 2015; Yang et al. 2015), and rurality (population density), residential instability, poverty, unemployment, and the percent of the population who are disabled and under the age of 65 were significantly related to the opioid prescribing rates (Guy et al. 2017; Heins et al. 2018; Stein et al. 2015). More importantly, the majority of these significant relationships (all except for poverty) maintained their independent and statistically significant association with the opioid prescribing rate when estimated simultaneously in a multivariable model, controlling for the other relevant characteristics.

This research presents a meaningful step in understanding the associations between community characteristics and opioid prescribing rates at the county-level. Local jurisdictions can use these results to target high-risk areas for interventions. For example, areas that disproportionately experience the community characteristics examined in this research can invest in programs aimed to educate clinicians on overprescribing (Kattan et al. 2016) or provide innovative treatment resources for patients that may be exposed to opioids. Moreover, while demographics and population characteristics are not likely to be altered at the county-level deliberately, local governments could aim to specifically target the housing, employment, and health characteristics associated with opioid prescribing rates, such as residential instability, poverty, unemployment, and early life disability rates, to potentially reduce a population's exposure to opioids and, in turn, potentially have an effect on opioid prescribing practices.

References

Allison, P. D. (1999). *Multiple regression: A primer*. Thousand Oaks: Pine Forge Press.

Back, S. E., Payne, R. L., Simpson, A. N., & Brady, K. T. (2010). Gender and prescription opioids: Findings from the National Survey on Drug Use and Health. *Addictive Behaviors, 35*(11), 1001–1007.

California Department of Justice (2018). *Controlled substance utilization review and evaluation system*. Retrieved from https://oag.ca.gov/cures.

California Department of Public Health (2018). *California opioid overdose surveillance dashboard*. Retrieved from https://discovery.cdph.ca.gov/CDIC/ODdash/

Curtis, L. H., Stoddard, J., Radeva, J. I., Hutchinson, S., Dans, P. E., Wright, A., Woosley, R. L., & Schulman, K. A. (2006). Geographic variation in the prescription of Schedule II opioid analgesics among outpatients in the United States. *Health Services Research, 41*, 837–855.

Guy, G. P., Jr., Zhang, K., Bohm, M. K., Losby, J., Lewis, B., Young, R., Murphy, L. B., & Dowell, D. (2017). Vital signs: Changes in opioid prescribing in the United States, 2006–2015. *Morbidity and Mortality Weekly Report, 66*(26), 697–704.

Heins, S. E., Sorbero, M. J., Jones, C. M., Dick, A. W., & Stein, B. A. (2018). High-risk prescribing to Medicaid enrollees receiving opioid analgesics: Individual and county-level factors. *Substance Abuse & Misuse, 53*, 1591–1601.

Hwang, C. S., Kang, E. M., Kornegay, C. J., Staffa, J. A., Jones, C. M., & McAninch, J. K. (2016). Trends in the concomitant prescribing of opioids and benzodiazepines, 2002–2014. *American Journal of Preventive Medicine, 51*(21), 151–160.

Joynt, M., Train, M. K., Robbins, B. W., Halterman, J. S., Caiola, E., & Fortuna, R. J. (2013). The impact of neighborhood socioeconomic status and race on the prescribing of opioids in emergency departments throughout the United States. *Journal of General Internal Medicine, 28*(12), 1604–1610.

Kattan, J. A., Tuazon, E., Paone, D., Dowell, D., Vo, L., Starrels, J. L., et al. (2016). Public health detailing—A successful strategy to promote judicious opioid analgesic prescribing. *American Journal of Public Health, 106*(8), 1430–1438.

Liu, Y., Logan, J. E., Paulozzi, L. J., Zhang, K., & Jones, C. M. (2013). Potential misuse and inappropriate prescription practices involving opioid analgesics. *The American Journal of Managed Care, 19*(8), 648–665.

National Institute on Drug Abuse (2018). *California opioid summary*. Retrieved from https://www.drugabuse.gov/drugs-abuse/opioids/opioid-summaries-by-state/california-opioid-summary.

Osgood, D. W. (2000). Poisson-based regression analysis of aggregate crime rates. *Journal of Quantitative Criminology, 16*, 21–43.

Paulozzi, L. J., Strickler, G. K., Kreiner, P. W., & Koris, C. M. (2015). Controlled substance prescribing patterns—Prescription behavior surveillance system, eight states, 2013. *MMWR Surveillance Summaries, 64*(9), 1–14.

Pletcher, M. J., Kertesz, S. G., Kohn, M. A., & Gonzales, R. (2008). Trends in opioid prescribing by race/ethnicity for patients seeking care in US emergency departments. *JAMA, 299*(1), 70–78.

Pratt, T. C., & Cullen, F. T. (2005). Assessing macro-level predictors and theories of crime: A meta-analysis. *Crime & Justice, 32*, 373–450.

Shaw, C. R., & McKay, H. D. (1942). *Juvenile delinquency and urban areas*. Chicago: University of Chicago Press.

Stein, B. D., Pacula, R. L., Gordon, A. J., Burns, R. M., Leslie, D. L., Sorbero, M. J., et al. (2015). Where is buprenorphine dispensed to treat opioid use disorders? The role of private offices, opioid treatment programs, and substance abuse treatment facilities in urban and rural counties. *Milbank Quarterly, 93*(3), 561–583.

U.S. Census Bureau (2017). *Quick facts: California*. Retrieved from https://www.census.gov/quickfacts/ca.

Yang, Z., Wilsey, B., Bohm, M., Weyrich, M., Roy, K., Ritley, D., et al. (2015). Defining risk of prescription opioid overdose: Pharmacy shopping & overlapping prescriptions among long-term opioid users in Medicaid. *The Journal of Pain, 16*(5), 445–453.

Chapter 4
Association Between Opioid Prescribing Rates and Criminal Justice Outcomes

The association between drugs and crime is quite complex and has been examined from a variety of perspectives in recent decades (McBride and McCoy 1993). Various studies have estimated the relationship between drug use (or the use of a specific drug) and both property crime and violent crime. Research has shown that drug abuse and predatory criminal activity often coexist, but the causal direction of this relationship is not clear (Chaiken and Chaiken 1990; Menard et al. 2001). Still, some studies have found that increases in drug use are associated with subsequent increases in crime (Horney et al.1995; Thompson and Uggen 2012).

One potential explanation for this may be that people who use drugs engage in economically motivated criminal activity to obtain money to support their drug use (Felson and Staff 2017). Another explanation may be that people who use drugs engage in violent crimes as a result of the pharmacological effects of the drug, including prescription drugs (Goldstein 1985; Molero et al. 2015). Other studies have examined the consequences of drug use and sales as predictors of crime. For example, Wendel et al. (2016) found that changes to the drug market might lead to decreases in crime.

While the aforementioned studies are relevant in that they consider the effects of drug use on criminal justice outcomes, such as criminal incidents and arrests, none have specifically examined the role of prescription opioid use on these outcomes. The societal costs of prescription opioid abuse are substantial, affecting the U.S. healthcare system, workplaces nationwide, as well as the criminal justice system. Using data from 2007, Birnbaum and colleagues (2011) estimated the societal costs of prescription opioid abuse. The research team estimated that criminal justice costs accounted for $5.1 billion in the United States (spent on police protection, legal and adjudication, correctional facilities, and property lost due to crime estimated to be associated with opioids). This amounted to about 9.2% of the total costs, estimated to be $55.7 billion (Birnbaum et al. 2011). While this data is over a

W. G. Jennings et al., *Opioid Prescribing Rates and Criminal Justice and Health Outcomes*, SpringerBriefs in Criminology,
https://doi.org/10.1007/978-3-030-40764-3_4

decade old, researchers remain unaware of the specific impact of the opioid prescribing rate on crime in the U.S.

4.1 Research Question 2

While prior research has examined some aspects of the opioid epidemic and public health outcomes, no empirical analysis has examined the effects of this crisis on criminal arrest rates at the county-level. As such, the current chapter will examine the associations between the opioid prescribing rate and three different offense arrest rates (violent crime, property crime, and drug crime) as well as the total arrest rate for each county in California. These associations will be examined in a multivariable framework in order to assess the relationship, while controlling for other relevant community characteristics (demographics, population density, housing, income, employment, and health).

4.2 Data Sources

In order to examine these relationships, three primary data sources were used: (1) U.S. Census Bureau (2017) data; (2) arrest data from California Department of Justice's (DOJ) Criminal Justice Statistics Center (CJSC); and (3) California's PBSS data (described in Chap. 2).

4.3 Dependent Variables

In order to examine various types of criminal behavior, four separate arrest rate outcome variables were generated for this analysis. First, a total annual arrest rate was generated for each county for 2012 through 2017 (per 100,000 residents). This included all violent crime arrests (homicide, rape, robbery, assault, and kidnapping), property crime arrests (burglary, theft, motor vehicle theft, forgery, and arson), and drug crime arrests (narcotics, marijuana, dangerous drugs, and other). Any other minor violations that resulted in an arrest were not included. Annual rates were averaged to create the mean arrest rate for each county from 2012 to 2017. Next, a separate annual arrest rate was generated for each type of crime (violent crime, property crime, and drug crime). Again, these annual arrest rates were averaged to create one mean-level rate for each crime type (per 100,000 residents). These four distinct measures allowed for the examination of the association of a county's opioid prescribing rates on the total crime rate as well as the association on each specific type of crime rate.

4.4 Opioid Prescribing Rate

The main independent variable of interest is the opioid prescribing rate for each county in California from 2012–2017 (as described in Chap. 3).

4.5 Community Characteristics

Obtained from the U.S. Census Bureau (2017) data, various community characteristics were also included in this analysis as control measures (as described in Chap. 3) such as demographics, population density, housing, income, employment, and health characteristics.

4.6 Analytic Strategy

To assess the association between the opioid prescribing rate and the rate of arrests in California counties from 2012–2017, two stages of analysis were performed using Stata 15.0. In the first stage of the analysis, descriptive statistics are reported for the opioid prescribing rate, arrest rates, and the community characteristics. In the second stage of the analysis, the association between the opioid prescribing rate and the arrest rates is examined in a series of four regression models. Since the dependent variables were represented as rates and due to the skewness observed in the distribution of the arrest rates, Poisson regression models were estimated producing standardized regression coefficients (Osgood 2000). Each Poisson regression model was estimated using identical independent variables and each of the four annual arrest rates from 2012–2017 (Total Crime, Violent Crime, Property Crime, and Drug Crime). In addition to the main variable of interest (opioid prescribing rate from 2012–2017), each model included all community characteristics (demographics, population density, housing, income, employment, and health).

4.7 Results

Table 4.1 presents the descriptive statistics of each of the community characteristics included in the analysis (n = 58). On average, percent female was 49.50% (SD = 2.12), percent White was 81.05% (SD = 10.62), and percent age 18 and younger was 22.05% (SD = 4.18). The average population per square mile was 663.25 (SD = 2314.75). The average residential stability was 84.97% (SD = 3.70) and the average poverty percentage was 15.13% (SD = 4.84). The average percentage of unemployed residents was 14.93% (SD = 4.12) and the average percentage of

Table 4.1 California county-level descriptive statistics demographic, population, housing, income, employment, and health characteristics and 2012–2017 opioid prescribing rates and 2012–2017 crime rates (n = 58)

Variables	M	SD	Minimum	Maximum
Demographic characteristics				
% Female	49.50	2.12	37.50	51.70
% White	81.05	10.62	50.20	93.90
% Age 18 and younger	22.05	4.18	13.40	30.90
Population characteristics				
Population per square mile	663.25	2314.75	1.60	17179.10
Housing characteristics				
% Residential stability	84.97	3.70	73.90	94.90
Income characteristics				
% Poverty	15.13	4.84	6.60	25.50
Employment characteristics				
% Unemployed	14.93	4.12	8.40	27.00
Health characteristics				
% Disabled under age 65	9.69	3.76	3.10	18.60
Opioid prescribing rates*				
Opioid prescribing rate (2012–2017)	221.86	80.93	64.12	1416.42
Crime rates**				
Total arrest rate (2012–2017)	867.39	273.06	488.22	2024.67
Violent arrest rate (2012–2017)	340.91	105.45	179.40	608.76
Property arrest rate (2012–2017)	245.08	70.77	118.53	428.01
Drug arrest rate (2012–2017)	281.40	157.13	130.42	1210.69

*Per 1000 residents
**Per 100,000 residents

disabled residents under the age of 65 was 9.69% (SD = 3.76). The mean county-level annual opioid prescribing rate from 2012–2017 was 221.86 (SD = 80.93).

Each of the four arrest rates is presented in Table 4.1 as well (per 100,000 residents). The average total arrest rate from 2012–2017 was 867.39 (SD = 273.06). Broken down into each category from 2012–2017, the average violent crime arrest rate was 340.91 (SD = 340.91), the average property crime arrest rate was 245.08 (SD = 70.77), and the average drug crime arrest rate was 281.40 (SD = 157.13).

Table 4.2 presents the standardized regression estimates of each of the four models. In the first model, the county-level opioid prescribing rate was significantly associated with the total crime arrest rate in California from 2012–2017 ($\beta = 1.133$, $p < 0.001$) adjusting for a number of other theoretically grounded community characteristics. In fact, each standard deviation increase in opioid prescribing rates was associated with a 13.3% increase in the total crime arrest rate. Beyond this relationship, percent 18 and younger ($\beta = 1.050$, $p < 0.001$), residential stability ($\beta = 1.055$, $p < 0.001$), poverty ($\beta = 1.059$, $p < 0.001$), percent unemployed ($\beta = 1.028$, $p < 0.001$), and percent disabled under the age of 65 ($\beta = 1.034$, $p < 0.001$) were all associated with the total crime arrest rate. On the other hand, percent identifying as

Table 4.2 Standardized regression estimates of the association between California county-level demographic, population, housing, income, employment, and health characteristics, 2012–2017 opioid prescribing rates, and 2012–2017 crime rates

Variables	Total crime arrest rate (2012–2017) Est. (% change)	Violent crime arrest rate (2012–2017) Est. (% change)	Property crime arrest rate (2012–2017) Est. (% change)	Drug crime arrest rate (2012–2017) Est. (% change)
Demographic characteristics				
% Female	1.002 (+0.2%)	0.952*** (-4.8%)	1.047*** (+4.7%)	1.032** (+3.2%)
% White	0.957*** (-4.3%)	0.945*** (-5.5%)	0.936*** (-6.4%)	1.011 (+1.1%)
% Age 18 and younger	1.050*** (+5.0%)	1.096*** (+9.6%)	1.177*** (+17.7%)	0.914*** (-8.6%)
Population characteristics				
Population per square mile	0.982** (-1.8%)	0.986 (-1.4%)	1.001 (+0.1%)	0.969* (-3.1%)
Housing characteristics				
% Residential stability	1.055*** (+5.5%)	1.081*** (+8.1%)	0.981 (-1.9%)	1.082*** (+8.2%)
Income characteristics				
% Poverty	1.159*** (+15.9%)	1.111*** (+11.1%)	1.047*** (+4.7%)	1.331*** (+33.1%)
Employment characteristics				
% Unemployed	1.028*** (+2.8%)	0.999 (-0.1%)	1.025* (+2.5%)	1.055*** (+5.5%)
Health characteristics				
% Disabled under age 65	1.034*** (+3.4%)	1.089*** (+8.9%)	1.079*** (+7.9%)	0.935*** (-6.5%)
Opioid prescribing rates				
Opioid Prescribing Rate (2012–2017)	1.133*** (+13.3%)	1.107*** (+10.7%)	1.087*** (+8.7%)	1.202*** (+20.2%)
-Log Likelihood= Pseudo R^2=	-886.18 0.64	-590.01 0.48	-411.87 0.47	-872.13 0.56

Est. = Estimates; estimates represent standardized Poisson regression coefficients
% Change reflects the percent increase/decrease in the crime rate for every standard deviation increase in the independent variable
*p < .05
**p < .01
***p < .001

White ($\beta = 0.950$, $p < 0.001$) and population per square mile ($\beta = 0.982$, $p < 0.01$) were both negatively associated with the total crime arrest rate. The association between sex composition and total crime arrest rates was not found to be significant in this model.

In the second model, the county-level opioid prescribing rate was again significantly associated with the violent crime arrest rate in California from 2012–2017 ($\beta = 1.107$, $p < 0.001$), despite controlling for other county-level factors. Each standard deviation increase in opioid prescribing rates was associated with a 10.7% increase in the violent crime arrest rate. Regarding the community characteristics in the model, mostly similar associations were found for the violent crime arrest rate as were identified for the total crime arrest rate. The only key differences were regarding percent female, which was significantly associated with lower violent crime arrest rates ($\beta = 0.952$, $p < 0.001$), and population per square mile and percent unemployed, which did not remain significant.

In the third model, the county-level opioid prescribing rate remained significantly associated with the property crime arrest rate in California from 2012–2017 ($\beta = 1.087$, $p < 0.001$). In this model, each standard deviation increase in opioid prescribing rates was associated with an 8.7% increase in the property crime arrest rate. Concerning the community characteristics in the model, relatively similar associations were found for the property crime arrest rate as were identified for the total crime arrest rate. The only key differences were regarding percent female, which was significantly associated with higher property crime arrest rates ($\beta = 1.047$, $p < 0.001$), and population per square mile and residential stability, which were no longer significant.

In the final model, the county-level opioid prescribing rate remained significantly associated with the drug crime arrest rate in California from 2012–2017 ($\beta = 1.202$, $p < 0.001$). In this model, each standard deviation increase in opioid prescribing rates was associated with a 20.2% increase in the drug crime arrest rate. The associations between the drug crime arrest rates and the community characteristics were again largely consistent with those identified for the total crime arrest rates, with a few exceptions. For example, percent female was significantly associated with higher drug crime arrest rates ($\beta = 1.032$, $p < 0.01$), and age 18 and younger ($\beta = 0.914$, $p < 0.001$) and percent disabled under the age of 65 ($\beta = 0.935$, $p < 0.001$) were significantly associated with lower drug crime arrest rates. Finally, percent of the population identifying as White was not significant in the model.

4.8 Summary

The current chapter examined the associations between the opioid prescribing rates in California and criminal arrest rates from 2012–2017. Specifically, this analysis estimated the association between the annual opioid prescribing rate and the violent crime arrest rates, property crime arrest rates, drug crime arrest rates, and total crime arrest rates, while controlling for other relevant community characteristics.

Following the analyses presented in this chapter, a number of conclusions can be drawn.

Most importantly, the findings revealed that the county-level opioid prescribing rate was significantly associated with all four county-level criminal arrest rates. Increases in the county-level opioid prescribing rate were associated with increases in arrests rates for violent crime, property crime, drug crime, and total crime, even when controlling for demographics, population density, housing, income, employment, and health characteristics.

To our knowledge, this analysis is the first of its kind to estimate the association between opioid prescribing rates and criminal justice outcomes at the county-level. The finding that a higher rate of opioid prescribing is associated with an increase to arrest rates suggests that the effects go well-beyond the realm of public health. Generally, this research supports the hypothesis that macro-level increases in opioid prescribing practices may lead to increases in criminal involvement; however, since this is a county-level analysis, one cannot conclude that people using opioids or living in counties with higher opioid availability are committing more crime nor can we definitively explain why this relationship exists. Similarly, another possible explanation for the positive relationship could also be due to the fact that those who use opioids are at a higher risk for victimization and this could be partly reflected in the increased crime rates. Though the exact cause for this association is beyond the scope of this current study, this research presents the novel finding that opioid prescribing behavior is associated with arrest rates at the county-level in California.

Based on the results presented in this chapter, one could presume that curtailing opioid prescribing practices could have important implications for crime at the county-level. For example, if opioid prevention initiatives were successfully implemented to reduce prescribing behaviors, local crime rates (violent, property, and drug) could be reduced as a result. This only further illustrates the potential far-reaching effects of interventions targeting opioid prescribing, even suggesting the broad utility of these interventions in addressing other adverse social issues, such as crime and other family issues (such as child removals from the home (Quast et al. 2018). In light of these potential associations, evidence-based interventions could garner greater local political capital and stronger public support for implementation. Given the personal and financial costs to counties and the wide-ranging effects of the opioid epidemic (Birnbaum et al. 2011), prevention efforts may present an exceedingly cost-effective alternative. The results presented here suggest that the opioid prescribing is not just a public health issue, but it also meaningfully influences the criminal justice system through arrests for violent behavior, property crime, drug crime, and overall criminal activity.

References

Birnbaum, H. G., White, A. G., Schiller, M., Waldman, T., Cleveland, J. M., & Roland, C. L. (2011). Societal costs of prescription opioid abuse, dependence, and misuse in the United States. *Pain Medicine, 12*(4), 657–667.

Chaiken, J. M., & Chaiken, M. R. (1990). Drugs & predatory crime. *Crime & Justice, 13*, 203–239.
Felson, R. B., & Staff, J. (2017). Committing economic crime for drug money. *Crime & Delinquency, 63*(4), 375–390.
Goldstein, P. J. (1985). The drugs/violence nexus: A tripartite conceptual framework. *Journal of Drug Issues, 15*(4), 493–506.
Horney, J., Osgood, D. W., & Marshall, I. H. (1995). Criminal careers in the short-term: Intra-individual variability in crime and its relation to local life circumstances. *American Sociological Review, 60*, 655–673.
McBride, D. C., & McCoy, C. B. (1993). The drugs-crime relationship: An analytical framework. *The Prison Journal, 73*(3), 257–278.
Menard, S., Mihalic, S., & Huizinga, D. (2001). Drugs and crime revisited. *Justice Quarterly, 18*(2), 269–299.
Molero, Y., Lichtenstein, P., Zetterqvist, J., Gumpert, C. H., & Fazel, S. (2015). Selective serotonin reuptake inhibitors and violent crime: A cohort study. *PLoS Medicine, 12*(9), e1001875.
Osgood, D. W. (2000). Poisson-based regression analysis of aggregate crime rates. *Journal of Quantitative Criminology, 16*, 21–43.
Quast, T., Storch, E. A., & Yampolskaya, S. (2018). Opioid prescription rates and child removals: Evidence from Florida. *Health Aff (Millwood), 37*(1), 134–139.
Thompson, M., & Uggen, C. (2012). Dealers, thieves, and the common determinants of drug and nondrug illegal earnings. *Criminology, 50*, 1057–1087.
U.S. Census Bureau (2017). *Quick facts: California.* Retrieved from https://www.census.gov/quickfacts/ca.
Wendel, T., Dhondt, G., Curtis, R., & Hamilton, J. (2016). "More drugs, less crime": Why crime dropped in New York City, 1985–2007. *Dialectical Anthropology, 40*(4), 319–339.

Chapter 5
Association Between Opioid Prescribing Rates and Health Outcomes

The harmful public health outcomes associated with opioid prescribing, including increased emergency department visits, hospitalizations, and overdose deaths, are well documented (Baumblatt et al. 2014; Braden et al. 2010; Dilokthornsakul et al. 2016; Ekstrom et al. 2014; Hall et al. 2008; Park et al. 2015; Spooner et al. 2016). Braden and colleagues (2010) found that people using opioids who experienced headaches, back pain, and pre-existing substance use disorders had a higher likelihood of emergency department visits. Additionally, their results suggested that some specific short-acting Drug Enforcement Agency (DEA) Schedule II opioids were associated with emergency department use when compared with other opioid types (Braden et al. 2010). Beyond the emergency department visits and hospitalizations, high-risk opioid use was examined as a predictor of overdose deaths as well.

Higher opioid dosage has been associated with an increased risk of opioid overdose death (Baumblatt et al. 2014; Bohnert et al. 2011; Dunn et al. 2010). For example, in a sample of patients who died as a result of an opioid-related overdose, Dunn and colleagues (2010) found that patients who received 1-20 mg had a 0.2% annual overdose rate, while patients who received 100 mg or more had a 1.8% annual overdose rate. This represented an 8.9 fold increase in risk (Dunn et al. 2010). Other high-risk opioid use patterns, such as patients who visit four or more prescribers or four or more pharmacies, were also associated with an increased risk for opioid-related overdose death (Baumblatt et al. 2014). Despite past research (see: Romeiser et al. 2019), these associations have not yet been estimated at the county-level for California to see if increases in opioid prescribing rates are associated with these opioid-related health outcomes.

W. G. Jennings et al., *Opioid Prescribing Rates and Criminal Justice and Health Outcomes*, SpringerBriefs in Criminology,
https://doi.org/10.1007/978-3-030-40764-3_5

5.1 Research Question 3

This chapter examines the associations between the annual opioid prescribing rate and three different opioid-related health outcomes (emergency room visit rates, hospitalization rates, and overdose rates) in California counties. These relationships were estimated using a multivariable model controlling for other relevant community characteristics (demographics, population density, housing, income, employment, and health).

5.2 Data Sources

In this analysis, three separate data sources were used: (1) U.S. Census Bureau (2017) data; (2) data from the California Opioid Overdose Surveillance Dashboard, which is a database that includes cause of death files provided by the California Department of Public Health (CDPH), emergency department visit and inpatient discharge data from the Office of Statewide Health Planning and Development (OSHPD); and (3) California PBSS data (described in Chap. 2).

5.3 Dependent Variables

Three separate outcome variables were generated for this analysis to examine various opioid-related health outcomes. First, a measure of the average rate of opioid-related emergency room visits was generated for each county from 2012–2017 (per 100,000 residents). This included all emergency department visits—regardless of intent (suicide, unintentional, or undetermined)—that were caused by non-fatal acute poisonings due to the effects of opioid drugs, excluding heroin. Emergency room visits due to the late or chronic effects of drugs (e.g. organ damage as a result of long-term use) were not included in this measure.

Next, a measure of the average rate of opioid-related hospitalizations was generated for each county from 2012–2016 (per 100,000 residents). This included any hospitalization caused by non-fatal acute poisonings due to the effects of opioid drugs, excluding heroin. Again, these visits were included in the data regardless of intent. Similar to the emergency room measure, hospitalizations due to the late or chronic effects of drugs were not included in this measure.

Finally, a measure of the average rate of opioid-related overdose deaths was generated for each county from 2012–2017 (per 100,000 residents). This outcome variable includes acute poisoning deaths that involved opioid pain relievers, heroin, and opium. Deaths that are related to the chronic use of these drugs were excluded from this measure.

5.4 Opioid Prescribing Rate

The main independent variable of interest is the opioid prescribing rate for each county in California from 2012–2017 (as described in Chap. 3).

5.5 Community Characteristics

A series of community characteristics (demographics, population density, housing, income, employment, and health) were included as control variables and were derived from the U.S. Census Bureau (2017) data (as described in Chap. 3).

5.6 Analytic Strategy

Three separate regression models were estimated using Stata 15.0 to assess the associations between the various independent variables and the outcome variables. Due to the fact that the dependent variables were represented as rates and skewed, Poisson regression models were estimated to generate standardized regression coefficients (Osgood 2000). Three regression models were estimated separately to examine the association between the opioid prescribing rate and each of the three opioid-related health outcomes (emergency room visits, hospitalizations, and overdose deaths). In addition to the main variable of interest (opioid prescribing rate from 2012–2017), each model included all of the community characteristics (demographics, population density, housing, income, employment, and health).

5.7 Results

Table 5.1 presents the descriptive statistics of each of the community characteristics included in the analysis (n = 58). On average, percent female was 49.50% (SD = 2.12), percent White was 81.05% (SD = 10.62), and percent age 18 and younger was 22.05% (SD = 4.18). The average population per square mile was 663.25 (SD = 2314.75). The average residential stability was 84.97% (SD = 3.70) and the average poverty percentage was 15.13% (SD = 4.84). The average percentage of unemployed residents was 14.93% (SD = 4.12) and the average percentage of disabled residents under the age of 65 was 9.69% (SD = 3.76). The mean county-level annual opioid prescribing rate from 2012–2017 was 221.86 (SD = 80.93).

Each of the three opioid-related health outcome rates is presented in Table 5.1 (per 1000 residents). The average county-level opioid-related emergency room visit rate from 2012–2017 was 16.42 (SD = 9.81). The average county-level

Table 5.1 California county-level descriptive statistics of demographic, population, housing, income, employment, and health characteristics and 2012–2017 opioid prescribing rates and opioid-related emergency room visit, hospitalization, and overdose rates (n = 58)

Variables	M	SD	Minimum	Maximum
Demographic characteristics				
% Female	49.50	2.12	37.50	51.70
% White	81.05	10.62	50.20	93.90
% Age 18 and younger	22.05	4.18	13.40	30.90
Population characteristics				
Population per square mile	663.25	2314.75	1.60	17179.10
Housing characteristics				
% Residential stability	84.97	3.70	73.90	94.90
Income characteristics				
% Poverty	15.13	4.84	6.60	25.50
Employment characteristics				
% Unemployed	14.93	4.12	8.40	27.00
Health characteristics				
% Disabled under age 65	9.69	3.76	3.10	18.60
Opioid prescribing rates				
Opioid prescribing rate (2012 –2017)	221.86	80.93	64.12	1416.42
Opioid-related health outcomes				
Opioid-related emergency room visit rate (2012–2017)	16.42	9.81	0.00	58.88
Opioid-related hospitalization rate (2012–2016)	14.72	9.53	0.00	48.78
Opioid-related overdose rate (2012–2017)	6.81	4.60	0.00	21.44

*Rates are per 1000 residents

opioid-related hospitalization rate from 2012–2016 was 14.72 (SD = 9.53). Finally, the average county-level opioid-related overdose death rate from 2012–2017 was 6.81 (SD = 4.60).

Table 5.2 presents the standardized regression estimates of the relationship between opioid prescribing rates and three negative opioid-related health outcomes (emergency room visit rate, hospitalization rate, and overdose rate) from 2012–2017 (2012–2016 for the hospitalization rate) while controlling for several community characteristics. In the first model, the county-level opioid prescribing rate was significantly associated with the opioid-related emergency room visit rate in California from 2012–2017 ($\beta = 1.120$, $p < 0.001$). This was found even after controlling for several community characteristics. Each standard deviation increase in opioid prescribing rates was associated with a 12.0% increase in the opioid-related emergency room visit rate. In addition to the opioid prescribing rate, percent identifying as White ($\beta = 1.098$, $p < 0.05$), population per square mile ($\beta = 1.125$, $p < 0.01$), percent unemployed ($\beta = 1.169$, $p < 0.01$), and percent disabled under the age of 65 ($\beta = 1.134$, $p < 0.001$) were all associated with a higher opioid-related emergency room visit rate. On the other hand, percent age 18 and younger was associated with a lower emergency room visit rate ($\beta = 0.878$, $p < 0.05$). Sex, residential stability,

Table 5.2 Standardized regression estimates of the association between california county-level demographic, population, housing, income, employment, and health characteristics and 2012–2017 opioid prescribing rates and opioid-related emergency room visit rates, hospitalization, and overdoses

Variables	Opioid-related emergency room visit rate (2012–2017) Est. (% change)	Opioid-related hospitalization rate (2012–2016) Est. (% change)	Opioid-related overdose rate (2012–2017) Est. (% change)
Demographic characteristics			
% Female	1.042 (+4.2%)	1.163** (+16.3%)	1.012 (+1.2%)
% White	1.098* (+9.8%)	1.166* (+16.6%)	1.086 (+8.6%)
% Age 18 and younger	0.878* (-12.2%)	1.124 (+12.4%)	0.787** (-22.3%)
Population characteristics			
Population per square mile	1.125** (+12.5%)	1.176** (+17.6%)	1.110 (+11.0%)
Housing characteristics			
% Residential stability	1.063 (+6.3%)	0.846*** (-15.4%)	0.884* (-11.6%)
Income characteristics			
% Poverty	1.060 (+6.0%)	0.956 (-3.4%)	1.167* (+16.7%)
Employment characteristics			
% Unemployed	1.169** (+16.9%)	0.971 (−2.9%)	1.168* (+16.8%)
Health characteristics			
% Disabled under age 65	1.134* (+13.4%)	1.078 (+7.8%)	0.791 (-20.9%)
Opioid prescribing rates			
Opioid prescribing rate (2012–2017)	1.120*** (+12.0%)	1.566*** (+56.6%)	1.497*** (+49.7%)
-Log Likelihood = Pseudo R^2=	-178.49 0.37	-161.25 0.42	-140.07 0.25

Est. = Estimates; estimates represent standardized Poisson regression coefficients
% Change reflects the percent increase/decrease in the opioid-related emergency room, hospitalization, or overdose rate for every standard deviation increase in the independent variable
*$p < .05$
**$p < .01$
***$p < .001$

and poverty were not associated with the opioid-related emergency room visit rate in this model.

In the second model, the county-level opioid prescribing rate was again significantly associated with the opioid-related hospitalization rate from 2012–2016 ($\beta = 1.566$, $p < 0.001$), despite controlling for other county-level factors. Each standard deviation increase in opioid prescribing rates was associated with a 56.6% increase in the opioid-related hospitalization rate. Regarding the community characteristics in the model, percent female ($\beta = 1.163$, $p < 0.01$), percent identifying as White ($\beta = 1.166$, $p < 0.05$), and population per square mile ($\beta = 1.176$, $p < 0.01$) were all associated with a higher opioid-related hospitalization rate. On the other hand, higher residential stability was associated with a lower opioid-related hospitalization rate ($\beta = 0.846$, $p < 0.001$). Age, poverty, unemployment, and disability under age 65 were not associated with the opioid-related hospitalization rate in this model.

In the final model, the county-level opioid prescribing rate was yet again significantly associated with the opioid-related overdose rate in California from 2012–2017 ($\beta = 1.497$, $p < 0.001$). For every one standard deviation increase in opioid prescribing rates, there was an associated 49.7% increase in the opioid-related overdose rate. Only poverty ($\beta = 1.167$, $p < 0.05$) and unemployment ($\beta = 1.168$, $p < 0.05$) were significantly associated with higher opioid-related overdose rates in this model. This may be the result of a lack of health insurance among those who are unemployed or living in poverty (for example, see Boscarino et al., 2016). Simultaneously, percent age 18 and younger ($\beta = 0.787$, $p < 0.01$) and residential stability ($\beta = 0.884$, $p < 0.05$) were associated with lower opioid-related overdose rates. All other variables in the model were non-significant.

5.8 Summary

This chapter examined the associations between the opioid prescribing rates in California and three opioid-related health outcomes from 2012–2017. Specifically, this analysis estimated the association between the annual opioid prescribing rate and emergency room visit rates, hospitalization rates, and overdose rates, while controlling for other relevant community characteristics. Key conclusions are outlined below.

The three regression models revealed that the county-level opioid prescribing rate was significantly associated with all three opioid-related health outcomes. An increase in the county-level opioid prescribing rate was associated with an increase in the opioid-related emergency room visit rate, hospitalization rate, and overdose rate, even when controlling for key community characteristics.

The current analysis supports past research indicating that opioid prescribing behavior is associated with several opioid-related adverse health outcomes (see: Baumblatt et al. 2014; Braden et al. 2010; Dilokthornsakul et al. 2016; Ekstrom et al. 2014; Hall et al. 2008; Park et al. 2015; Spooner et al. 2016). However, this is the first study to substantiate this relationship in counties in California. Given this is a county-level analysis, one cannot definitively conclude that opioid prescription recipients are the ones being admitted to the emergency room, hospitalized, or overdosing. We can assume, however, that higher levels of opioid prescribing behavior plays a major role in these opioid-related health outcomes.

Based on these findings, monitoring and reducing opioid prescribing practices could significantly reduce the rates of opioid-related emergency room visits, hospitalizations, and overdoses, alleviating some the burden on a county's healthcare system. Given that counties with higher opioid-prescribing rates were demonstrated to have higher rates of these adverse health outcomes, curbing these prescribing practices could provide reductions in the personal and financial costs of these opioid-related consequences. Again, a better recognition of these potential effects could help illustrate the necessity of initiatives aimed at monitoring and reducing the over-prescribing of opioids. Considering the strength of the relationship between the opioid-prescribing rate and hospitalizations and overdoses in particular, prevention practices could be the difference between life and death.

References

Baumblatt, J. A. G., Wiedeman, C., Dunn, J. R., Schaffner, W., Paulozzi, L. J., & Jones, T. F. (2014). High-risk use by patients prescribed opioids for pain and its role in overdose deaths. *JAMA Internal Medicine, 174*(5), 796–801.

Bohnert, A. S., Valenstein, M., Bair, M. J., Ganoczy, D., McCarthy, J. F., Ilgen, M. A., & Blow, F. C. (2011). Association between opioid prescribing patterns and opioid overdose-related deaths. *JAMA, 305*(13), 1315–1321.

Boscarino, J. A., Kirchner, H. L., Pitcavage, J. M., Nadipelli, V. R., Ronquest, N. A., Fitzpatrick, M. H., & Han, J. J. (2016). Factors associated with opioid overdose: a 10-year retrospective study of patients in a large integrated health care system. *Substance Abuse and Rehabilitation, 7*, 131–141.

Braden, J. B., Russo, J., Fan, M.-Y., Edlund, M. J., Martin, B. C., DeVries, A., & Sullivan, M. D. (2010). Emergency department visits among recipients of chronic opioid therapy. *Archives of Internal Medicine, 170*(16), 1425–1432.

Dilokthornsakul, P., Moore, G., Campbell, J. D., Lodge, R., Traugott, C., Zerzan, J., et al. (2016). Risk factors of prescription opioid overdose among Colorado Medicaid beneficiaries. *The Journal of Pain, 17*(4), 436–443.

Dunn, K. M., Saunders, K. W., Rutter, C. M., Banta-Green, C. J., Merrill, J. O., Sullivan, M. D., et al. (2010). Overdose and prescribed opioids: Associations among chronic non-cancer pain patients. *Annals of Internal Medicine, 152*(2), 85.

Ekstrom, M. P., Bornefalk-Hermansson, A., Abernethy, A. P., & Currow, D. C. (2014). Safety of benzodiazepines and opioids in very severe respiratory disease: National prospective study. *BMJ (Clinical Research Ed.), 348*, g445.

Hall, A. J., Logan, J. E., Toblin, R. L., Kaplan, J. A., Kraner, J. C., Bixler, D., et al. (2008). Patterns of abuse among unintentional pharmaceutical overdose fatalities. *Journal of the American Medical Association, 300*(22), 2613–2620.

Osgood, D. W. (2000). Poisson-based regression analysis of aggregate crime rates. *Journal of Quantitative Criminology, 16*, 21–43.

Park, T. W., Saitz, R., Ganoczy, D., Ilgen, M. A., & Bohnert, A. S. B. (2015). Benzodiazepine prescribing patterns and deaths from drug overdose among U.S. veterans receiving opioid analgesics: Case-cohort study. *BMJ (Clinical Research Ed.), 350*, h2698.

Romeiser, J. L., Labriola, J., & Meliker, J. R. (2019). Geographic patterns of prescription opioids and opioid overdose deaths in New York State, 2013–2015. *Drug and Alcohol Dependence, 195*, 94–100.

Spooner, L., Fernandes, K., Martins, D., Juurlink, D., Mamdani, M., Paterson, J. M., et al. (2016). High-dose opioid prescribing and opioid-related hospitalization: a population-based study. *PloS one, 11*(12), e0167479.

U.S. Census Bureau (2017). *Quick facts: California.* Retrieved from https://www.census.gov/quickfacts/ca.

Chapter 6
Conclusions

Nearly one in five Americans are prescribed an opioid each year (U.S. Centers for Disease Control and Prevention 2017a,b). Although opioid prescribing is generally found to be lower in California than nationwide, county-level prescribing and the outcomes associated with it are still worthy of thorough examination. This book utilized county-level opioid prescribing data in California from 2012–2017 to examine this problem in several ways. First, by summarizing the general trends in opioid prescribing from 2012–2017. Second, by examining the associations between community characteristics (demographics, population density, housing, income, employment, and health characteristics) and the opioid prescribing rate. Next, by estimating the association between the opioid prescribing rate and county-level arrest rates (violent, property, drug, and total crimes). And last, by assessing the association between the county-level opioid prescribing rates and three county-level opioid-related public health outcome rates, including emergency room visit rates, hospitalization rates, and overdose rates. The main findings of this project are outlined below.

6.1 Main Findings

Opioids were prescribed at a much higher rate from 2012 to 2017 as compared to stimulants and benzodiazepines. The overall California opioid prescribing rate decreased from 2012 to 2017 and many counties experienced a similar decline during the study period. Opioid prescribing rates declined for both males and females, but this decrease was more widespread for females than males. Furthermore, opioids were prescribed to older patients more often than younger patients. Hydrocodone SA was the most commonly prescribed opioid. All opioid prescribing rates, with the exception of Oxycodone SA, decreased from 2012 to 2017. In general, the mean

W. G. Jennings et al., *Opioid Prescribing Rates and Criminal Justice and Health Outcomes*, SpringerBriefs in Criminology,
https://doi.org/10.1007/978-3-030-40764-3_6

daily doses for all six of the most commonly prescribed opioids also declined. Opioid naïve patients were found to receive a smaller proportion of the overall prescriptions in 2017 than in 2012, but the top 1% of opioid prescribers wrote a larger percentage of opioid prescriptions.

Related to Research Question 1, the analysis revealed that each category of community characteristics (demographics, population density, housing, income, employment, and health characteristics) were independently and significantly associated with the 2012–2017 opioid prescribing rate. Counties with a higher percentage of females, people identifying as White, and older persons were associated with higher opioid prescribing rates. Rurality, residential instability, poverty, unemployment, and the percentage of the population who are disabled and under the age of 65 were also associated with increases in the opioid prescribing rate.

Related to Research Question 2, the county-level opioid prescribing rate was significantly associated with all four county-level criminal arrest rates (violent, property, drug, and total crime arrest rates). Higher county-level opioid prescribing rates were associated with higher levels of all four arrests rates, even when controlling for the community characteristics (see Appendix 2 for additional resources related to opioids and criminal justice).

Finally, related to Research Question 3, the county-level opioid prescribing rate was significantly associated with all three opioid-related public health outcomes (emergency room visit, hospitalization, and overdose rates). Higher county-level opioid prescribing rates were associated with higher levels of the each of the three opioid-related public health outcomes, even when controlling for the aforementioned community characteristics (see Appendix 2 for additional resources related to opioids and public health).

6.2 Policy Implications

These research findings suggest various implications for policy and clinical practice. Predominantly, this project emphasizes the importance of continued data collection and analysis on opioid prescribing at the local, state, and national level. Without the PBSS data, the analyses presented in this book are not possible, but the future of the PBSS as a national asset is uncertain. Furthermore, this project has taken a pivotal step in understanding potential community characteristics for opioid prescribing. While high-risk opioid prescribing and the associated negative public health outcomes were present in all 58 counties in California, these outcomes were not experienced uniformly. Some counties had prescribing rates that were several times higher than others. For example, in 2017, Lake County's opioid prescribing rate was more than four-times larger than in Alpine County. Based on these results, counties with elevated opioid prescribing rates should utilize more resources to educate prescribers about overprescribing to curb prescribing behaviors. Addressing some of the community characteristics for higher opioid prescribing rates, such as residential instability, poverty, unemployment, and early life disability rates, could also provide a fruitful avenue for reducing opioid prescribing.

Based on the results presented in this book, continuing to reduce California's prescribing trends, as recommended by the U.S. Department of Health and Human Services (2019), could positively impact both crime and public health issues at the county-level. For example, if prescribing rates were further controlled, crime rates and opioid-related hospital use and overdose rates could be reduced as a result. These analyses suggest a multitude of deleterious outcomes experienced by local communities as a result of the opioid crisis. Furthermore, these results suggest that prevention and reduction efforts targeting opioid prescribing could be effective in addressing various adverse social issues. Considering the costs of these adverse social issues to local communities, prevention programs may be a cost-effective way to alleviate the pain and deaths caused by high-risk opioid prescribing and the financial burden on the healthcare and criminal justice systems (Aroke et al. 2018; Birnbaum et al. 2011; Chang et al. 2018; Zajac et al. 2019). Ultimately, the opioid crisis cannot just be seen as a public health issue, but instead an issue affecting multiple systems and requiring a multi-disciplinary approach to be most effective.

6.3 Conclusion

The consequences of the opioid crisis are pervasive and in some cases severe; however, they are not experienced by all California counties equally. There are several negative consequences associated with the opioid crisis, such as criminal arrests, patient hospitalizations, emergency room visits, and overdose deaths, and communities more severely impacted by the opioid crisis may experience a culmination of negative outcomes with high costs. While several cities and states have attempted to address these costs through lawsuits against opioid manufacturers (see: NPR 2019), the mitigation of the personal consequences is impossible. Only through evidence-based prevention strategies can the opioid crisis be addressed and targeted at the local level.

References

Aroke, H., Buchanan, A., Wen, X., Ragosta, P., Koziol, J., & Kogut, S. (2018). Estimating the direct costs of outpatient opioid prescriptions: A retrospective analysis of data from the Rhode Island prescription drug monitoring program. *Journal of Managed Care & Specialty Pharmacy, 24*(3), 214–224.

Birnbaum, H. G., White, A. G., Schiller, M., Waldman, T., Cleveland, J. M., & Roland, C. L. (2011). Societal costs of prescription opioid abuse, dependence, and misuse in the United States. *Pain Medicine, 12*(4), 657–667.

Chang, H. Y., Kharrazi, H., Bodycombe, D., Weiner, J. P., & Alexander, G. C. (2018). Healthcare costs and utilization associated with high-risk prescription opioid use: A retrospective cohort study. *BMC Medicine, 16*(1), 69–80.

NPR (2019). Your guide to the massive (and massively complex) opioid litigation. Retrieved from https://www.npr.org/sections/health-shots/2019/10/15/761537367/your-guide-to-the-massive-and-massively-complex-opioid-litigation

U.S. Centers for Disease Control and Prevention (2017a). *Prescription opioid data.* U.S. Department of Health and Human Services. Retrieved from https://www.cdc.gov/drugoverdose/data/prescribing.html.

U.S. Centers for Disease Control and Prevention (2017b). *2018 Annual surveillance report of drug-related risks and outcomes.* U.S. Department of Health and Human Services. Retrieved from https://www.cdc.gov/drugoverdose/pdf/pubs/2018-cdc-drug-surveillance-report.pdf.

U.S. Department of Health and Human Services (2019). *HHS guide for clinicians on the appropriate dosage reduction or discontinuation of long-term opioid analgesics.* Retrieved from https://www.hhs.gov/opioids/sites/default/files/2019-10/Dosage_Reduction_Discontinuation.pdf

Zajac, G., Nur, S. A., Kreager, D. A., & Sterner, G. (2019). Estimated costs to the Pennsylvania criminal justice system resulting from the opioid crisis. *The American Journal of Managed Care, 25*(13), S250–S255.

Appendix 1: Supplemental Figures

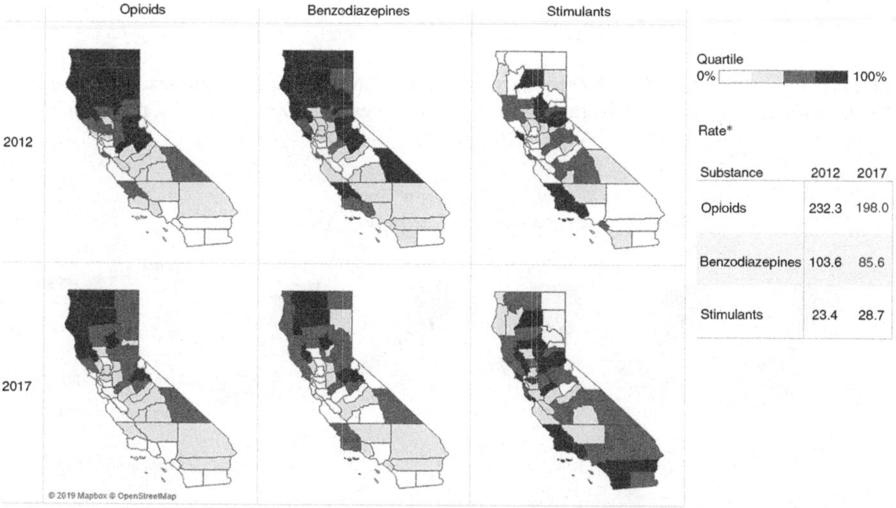

Fig. 1.1 Prescribing rates (per 1000 county population) by drug class, 2012 and 2017
Note: Yearly rate refers to the average of the quarterly rates per 1000 county population. Drug-specific quartiles created using pooled data for 2012 and 2017

W. G. Jennings et al., *Opioid Prescribing Rates and Criminal Justice and Health Outcomes*, SpringerBriefs in Criminology,
https://doi.org/10.1007/978-3-030-40764-3

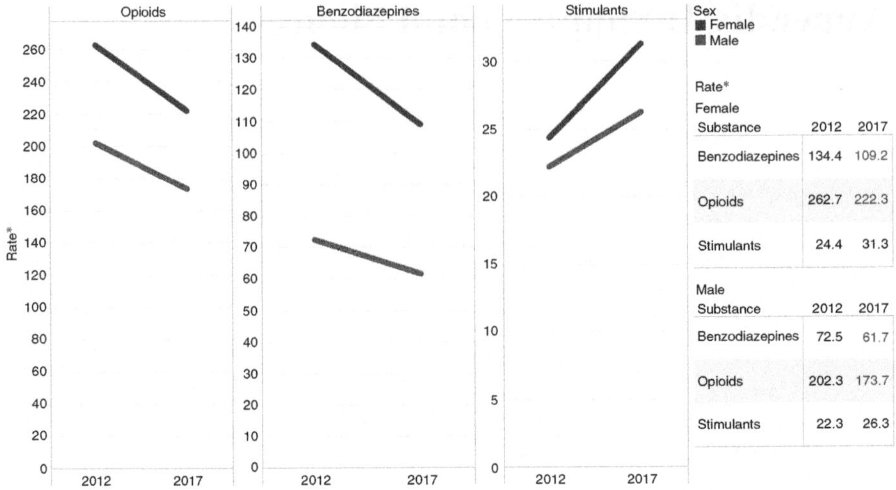

Fig. 1.2 Prescribing rates (per 1000 county-sex population) by drug class and sex, 2012 and 2017
Note: Yearly rate refers to the average of the quarterly rates per 1,000 county-sex population

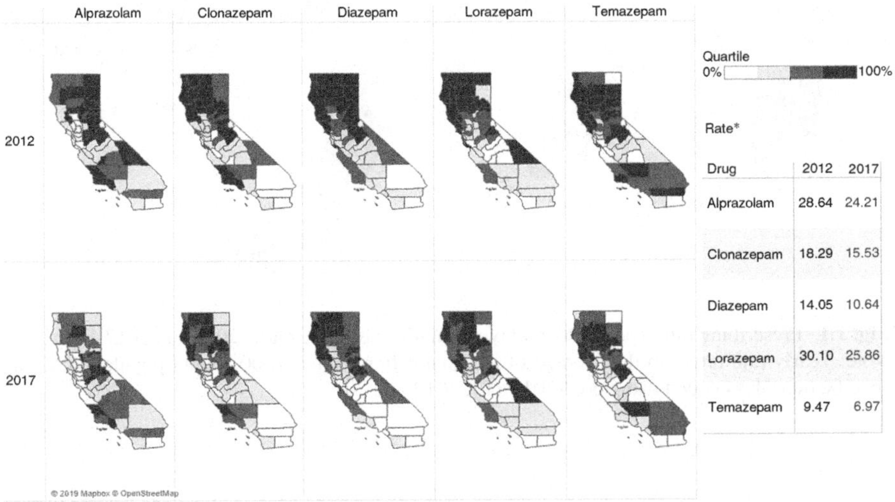

Fig. 1.3 Prescribing rates (per 1000 county population) by select benzodiazepine, 2012 and 2017
Note: Yearly rate refers to the average of the quarterly rates per 1000 county population. Drug-specific quartiles created using pooled data for 2012 and 2017

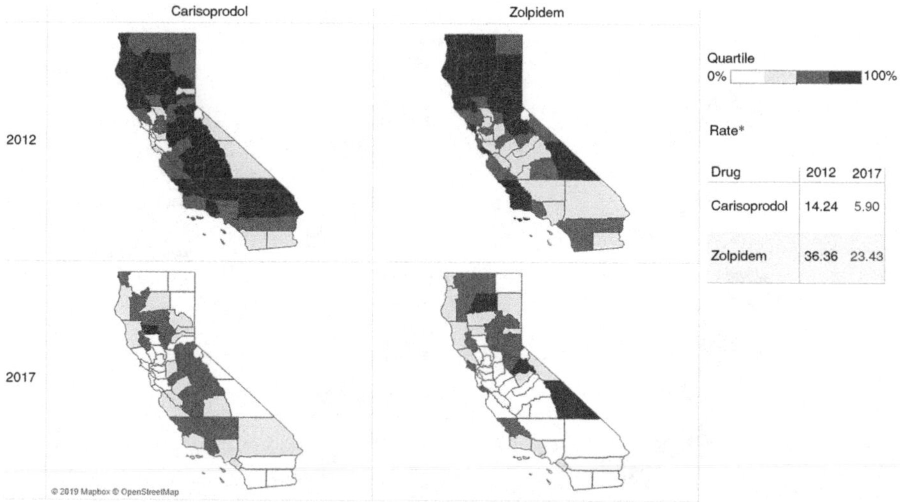

Fig. 1.4 Prescribing rates (per 1000 county population) for carisoprodol and Zolpidem, 2012 and 2017
Note: Yearly rate refers to the average of the quarterly rates per 1000 county population. Drug-specific quartiles created using pooled data for 2012 and 2017

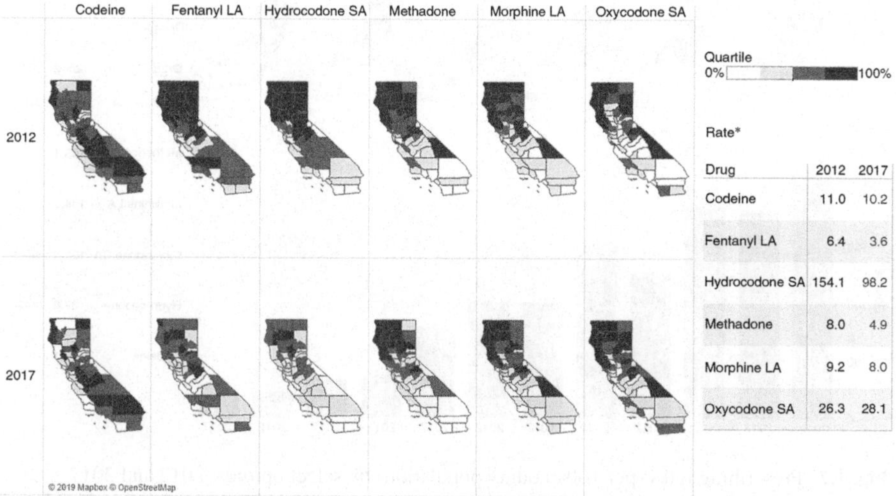

Fig. 1.5 Prescribing rates (per 1000 county population) by select opioid, 2012 and 2017
Note: Yearly rate refers to the average of the quarterly rates per 1000 county population. Drug-specific quartiles created using pooled data for 2012 and 2017

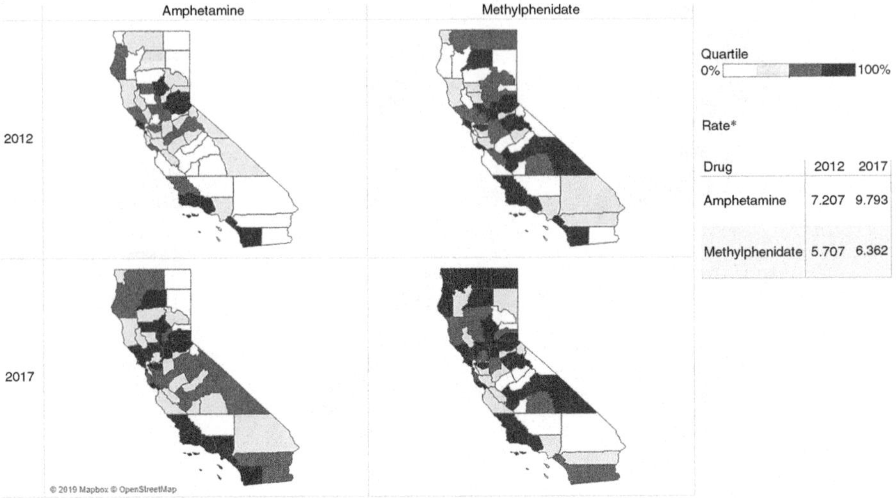
Amphetamine
Methylphenidate
2012
2017
Quartile
0%
100%
Rate*
Drug 2012 2017
Amphetamine 7.207 9.793
Methylphenidate 5.707 6.362
© 2019 Mapbox © OpenStreetMap

Fig. 1.6 Prescribing rates (per 1000 county population) by select stimulants, 2012 and 2017
Note: Yearly rate refers to the average of the quarterly rates per 1000 county population. Drug-specific quartiles created using pooled data for 2012 and 2017

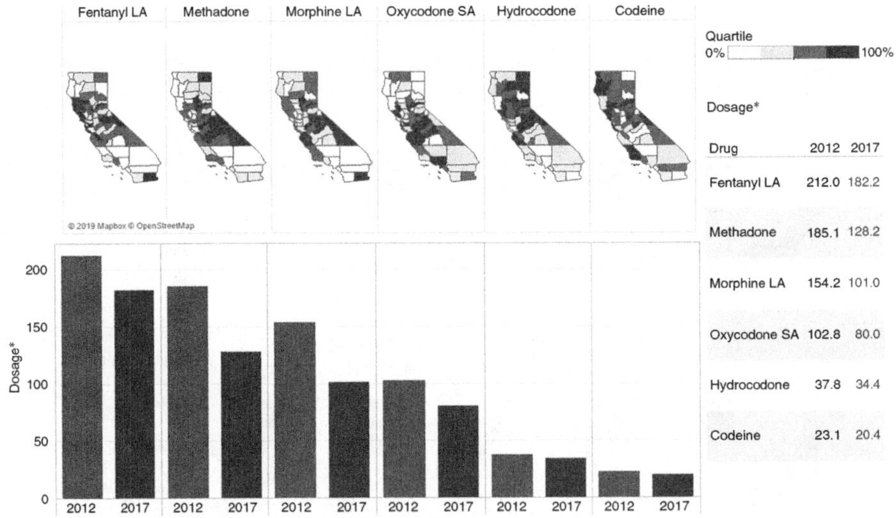

Fig. 1.7 Prescribing rates (per 1000 county population) by select opioids, 2012 and 2017
Note: Yearly rate refers to the average of the quarterly rates per 1000 county population. Drug-specific quartiles created using pooled data for 2012 and 2017. Dosage refers to averaged quarterly mean daily dosages per patient in morphine milligram equivalent

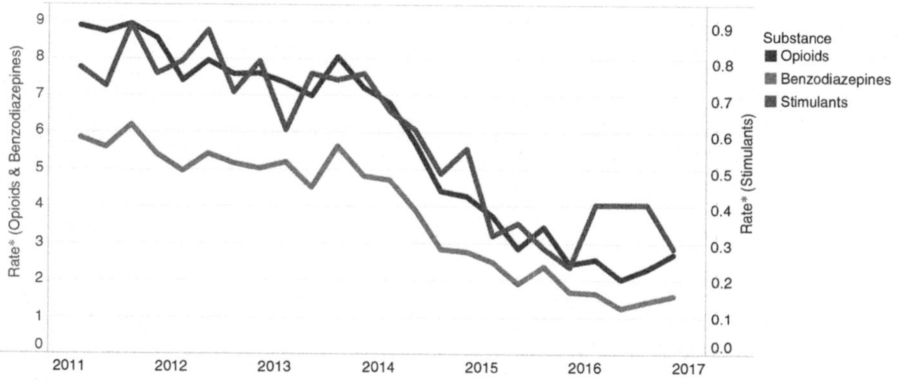

Yearly Rate*

Substance	2012	2013	2014	2015	2016	2017
Opioids	8.79	7.64	7.40	5.31	3.13	2.41
Benzodiazepines	5.77	5.15	5.05	3.56	2.12	1.48
Stimulants	0.81	0.81	0.73	0.59	0.31	0.38

Fig. 1.8 Multiple provider episode rates (per 1000 county population), by drug class, 2011–2017
Note: Yearly rate refers to the average of the quarterly rates per 1,000 county population

Appendix 2: Additional Readings

Al-Tayyib, A. A., Koester, S., & Riggs, P. (2017). Prescription opioids prior to injection drug use: Comparisons and public health implications. *Addictive Behaviors, 65*, 224–228.

Alexander, G. C., Kruszewski, S. P., & Webster, D. W. (2012). Rethinking opioid prescribing to protect patient safety and public health. *JAMA, 308*(18), 1865–1866.

Back, S. E., Payne, R. L., Simpson, A. N., & Brady, K. T. (2010). Gender and prescription opioids: Findings from the national survey on drug use and health. *Addictive Behaviors, 35*(11), 1001–1007.

Bailey, R. W., & Vowles, K. E. (2015). Chronic noncancer pain and opioids: Risks, benefits, and the public health debate. *Professional Psychology: Research and Practice, 46*(5), 340.

Banerjee, G., Edelman, E. J., Barry, D. T., Becker, W. C., Cerdá, M., Crystal, S., et al. (2016). Non-medical use of prescription opioids is associated with heroin initiation among US veterans: A prospective cohort study. *Addiction, 111*(11), 2021–2031.

Baumblatt, J. A. G., Wiedeman, C., Dunn, J. R., Schaffner, W., Paulozzi, L. J., & Jones, T. F. (2014). High-risk use by patients prescribed opioids for pain and its role in overdose deaths. *JAMA Internal Medicine, 174*(5), 796–801.

Becker, W. C., Sullivan, L. E., Tetrault, J. M., Desai, R. A., & Fiellin, D. A. (2008). Non-medical use, abuse and dependence on prescription opioids among US adults: Psychiatric, medical and substance use correlates. *Drug and Alcohol Dependence, 94*(1–3), 38–47.

Binswanger, I. A., & Glanz, J. M. (2015). Pharmaceutical opioids in the home and youth: Implications for adult medical practice. *Substance Abuse, 36*(2), 141–143.

Binswanger, I. A., Koester, S., Mueller, S. R., Gardner, E. M., Goddard, K., & Glanz, J. M. (2015). Overdose education and naloxone for patients prescribed opioids in primary care: A qualitative study of primary care staff. *Journal of General Internal Medicine, 30*(12), 1837–1844.

Birnbaum, H. G., White, A. G., Reynolds, J. L., Greenberg, P. E., Zhang, M., Vallow, S., et al. (2006). Estimated costs of prescription opioid analgesic abuse in the United States in 2001: A societal perspective. *The Clinical Journal of Pain, 22*(8), 667–676.

Birnbaum, H. G., White, A. G., Schiller, M., Waldman, T., Cleveland, J. M., & Roland, C. L. (2011). Societal costs of prescription opioid abuse, dependence, and misuse in the United States. *Pain Medicine, 12*(4), 657–667.

W. G. Jennings et al., *Opioid Prescribing Rates and Criminal Justice and Health Outcomes*, SpringerBriefs in Criminology,
https://doi.org/10.1007/978-3-030-40764-3

Black, R. A., Trudeau, K. J., Cassidy, T. A., Budman, S. H., & Butler, S. F. (2013). Associations between public health indicators and injecting prescription opioids by prescription opioid abusers in substance abuse treatment. *Journal of Opioid Management, 9*(1), 5–17.

Brinkley-Rubinstein, L., Zaller, N., Martino, S., Cloud, D. H., McCauley, E., Heise, A., & Seal, D. (2018). Criminal justice continuum for opioid users at risk of overdose. *Addictive Behaviors, 86*, 104–110.

Bukten, A., Skurtveit, S., Stangeland, P., Gossop, M., Willersrud, A. B., Waal, H., et al. (2011). Criminal convictions among dependent heroin users during a 3-year period prior to opioid maintenance treatment: A longitudinal national cohort study. *Journal of Substance Abuse Treatment, 41*(4), 407–414.

Burgess, D. J., Crowley-Matoka, M., Phelan, S., Dovidio, J. F., Kerns, R., Roth, C., et al. (2008). Patient race and physicians' decisions to prescribe opioids for chronic low back pain. *Social Science & Medicine, 67*(11), 1852–1860.

Byford, S., Barrett, B., Metrebian, N., Groshkova, T., Cary, M., Charles, V., et al. (2013). Cost-effectiveness of injectable opioid treatment v. oral methadone for chronic heroin addiction. *The British Journal of Psychiatry, 203*(5), 341–349.

Campbell, G., Hall, W. D., Peacock, A., Lintzeris, N., Bruno, R., Larance, B., et al. (2018). Effect of cannabis use in people with chronic non-cancer pain prescribed opioids: Findings from a 4-year prospective cohort study. *The Lancet: Public Health, 3*(7), e341–e350.

Centers for Disease Control and Prevention (CDC). (2012). Vital signs: Risk for overdose from methadone used for pain relief-United States, 1999–2010. *MMWR. Morbidity and Mortality Weekly Report, 61*(26), 493.

Centers for Disease Control and Prevention. (2016). Guideline for prescribing opioids for chronic pain. *Journal of Pain & Palliative Care Pharmacotherapy, 30*(2), 138–140.

Chandler, R. K., Finger, M. S., Farabee, D., Schwartz, R. P., Condon, T., Dunlap, L. J., et al. (2016). The SOMATICS collaborative: Introduction to a National Institute on drug abuse cooperative study of pharmacotherapy for opioid treatment in criminal justice settings. *Contemporary Clinical Trials, 48*, 166–172.

Chen, J. H., Humphreys, K., Shah, N. H., & Lembke, A. (2016). Distribution of opioids by different types of medicare prescribers. *JAMA Internal Medicine, 176*(2), 259–261.

Cherny, N. I., Baselga, J., De Conno, F., & Radbruch, L. (2010). Formulary availability and regulatory barriers to accessibility of opioids for cancer pain in Europe: A report from the ESMO/EAPC opioid policy initiative. *Annals of Oncology, 21*(3), 615–626.

Chinellato, A., Terrazzani, G., Walley, T., & Giusti, P. (2003). Opioids in Italy: Is marketing more powerful than the law? *The Lancet, 362*(9377), 78.

Chou, R., Turner, J. A., Devine, E. B., Hansen, R. N., Sullivan, S. D., Blazina, I., et al. (2015). The effectiveness and risks of long-term opioid therapy for chronic pain: A systematic review for a National Institutes of health pathways to prevention workshop. *Annals of Internal Medicine, 162*(4), 276–286.

Clark, C. B., Hendricks, P. S., Lane, P. S., Trent, L., & Cropsey, K. L. (2014). Methadone maintenance treatment may improve completion rates and delay opioid relapse for opioid dependent individuals under community corrections supervision. *Addictive Behaviors, 39*(12), 1736–1740.

Cleary, J., Powell, R. A., Munene, G., Mwangi-Powell, F. N., Luyirika, E., Kiyange, F., et al. (2013). Formulary availability and regulatory barriers to accessibility of opioids for cancer pain in Africa: A report from the Global Opioid Policy Initiative (GOPI). *Annals of Oncology, 24*(suppl_11), xi14–xi23.

Coe, M. A., Pillitteri, J. L., Sembower, M. A., Gerlach, K. K., & Henningfield, J. E. (2019). Kratom as a substitute for opioids: Results from an online survey. *Drug and Alcohol Dependence, 202*, 24–32.

Coviello, D. M., Cornish, J. W., Lynch, K. G., Alterman, A. I., & O'Brien, C. P. (2010). A randomized trial of oral naltrexone for treating opioid-dependent offenders. *The American Journal on Addictions, 19*(5), 422–432.

Coviello, D. M., Cornish, J. W., Lynch, K. G., Boney, T. Y., Clark, C. A., Lee, J. D., et al. (2012). A multisite pilot study of extended-release injectable naltrexone treatment for previously opioid-dependent parolees and probationers. *Substance Abuse, 33*(1), 48–59.

Cropsey, K. L., Lane, P. S., Hale, G. J., Jackson, D. O., Clark, C. B., Ingersoll, K. S., et al. (2011). Results of a pilot randomized controlled trial of buprenorphine for opioid dependent women in the criminal justice system. *Drug and Alcohol Dependence, 119*(3), 172–178.

Dale, O., Borchgrevink, P. C., Fredheim, O. M. S., Mahic, M., Romundstad, P., & Skurtveit, S. (2015). Prevalence of use of non-prescription analgesics in the Norwegian HUNT3 population: Impact of gender, age, exercise and prescription of opioids. *BMC Public Health, 15*(1), 461.

Dasgupta, N., Freifeld, C., Brownstein, J. S., Menone, C. M., Surratt, H. L., Poppish, L., et al. (2013). Crowdsourcing black market prices for prescription opioids. *Journal of Medical Internet Research, 15*(8), e178.

Dasgupta, N., Kramer, E. D., Zalman, M. A., Carino, S., Jr., Smith, M. Y., Haddox, J. D., & Wright, C., IV. (2006). Association between non-medical and prescriptive usage of opioids. *Drug and Alcohol Dependence, 82*(2), 135–142.

Degenhardt, L., Bucello, C., Mathers, B., Briegleb, C., Ali, H., Hickman, M., & McLaren, J. (2011). Mortality among regular or dependent users of heroin and other opioids: A systematic review and meta-analysis of cohort studies. *Addiction, 106*(1), 32–51.

Degenhardt, L., Gisev, N., Trevena, J., Larney, S., Kimber, J., Burns, L., et al. (2013). Engagement with the criminal justice system among opioid-dependent people: A retrospective cohort study. *Addiction, 108*(12), 2152–2165.

Deyo, R. A., Von Korff, M., & Duhrkoop, D. (2015). Opioids for low back pain. *BMJ, 350*, g6380.

Dublin, S., Walker, R. L., Jackson, M. L., Nelson, J. C., Weiss, N. S., Von Korff, M., & Jackson, L. A. (2011). Use of opioids or benzodiazepines and risk of pneumonia in older adults: A population-based case–control study. *Journal of the American Geriatrics Society, 59*(10), 1899–1907.

Ducharme, L. J., & Roman, P. M. (2009). Opioid treatment programs in the clinical trials network: Representativeness and buprenorphine adoption. *Journal of Substance Abuse Treatment, 37*(1), 90–94.

Edlund, M. J., Martin, B. C., Devries, A., Fan, M. Y., Braden, J. B., & Sullivan, M. D. (2010). Trends in use of opioids for chronic non-cancer pain among individuals with mental health and substance use disorders: The TROUP study. *The Clinical Journal of Pain, 26*(1), 1–8.

Edlund, M. J., Steffick, D., Hudson, T., Harris, K. M., & Sullivan, M. (2007). Risk factors for clinically recognized opioid abuse and dependence among veterans using opioids for chronic non-cancer pain. *Pain, 129*(3), 355–362.

Edwards, H. E., Nash, R. E., Najman, J. M., Yates, P. M., Fentiman, B. J., Dewar, A., et al. (2001). Determinants of nurses' intention to administer opioids for pain relief. *Nursing & Health Sciences, 3*(3), 149–159.

Edwards, R. R., Wasan, A. D., Michna, E., Greenbaum, S., Ross, E., & Jamison, R. N. (2011). Elevated pain sensitivity in chronic pain patients at risk for opioid misuse. *The Journal of Pain, 12*(9), 953–963.

Finlay, A. K., Harris, A. H., Rosenthal, J., Blue-Howells, J., Clark, S., McGuire, J., et al. (2016). Receipt of pharmacotherapy for opioid use disorder by justice-involved US veterans health administration patients. *Drug and Alcohol Dependence, 160*, 222–226.

Fischer, B., & Rehm, J. (2008). Nonmedical use of prescription opioids: Furthering a meaningful research agenda. *The Journal of Pain, 9*(6), 490–493.

Fischer, B., Goldman, B., Rehm, J., & Popova, S. (2008). Non-medical use of prescription opioids and public health in Canada. *Canadian Journal of Public Health, 99*(3), 182–184.

Fischer, B., Keates, A., Bühringer, G., Reimer, J., & Rehm, J. (2014). Non-medical use of prescription opioids and prescription opioid-related harms: Why so markedly higher in North America compared to the rest of the world? *Addiction, 109*(2), 177–181.

Fischer, B., Lusted, A., Roerecke, M., Taylor, B., & Rehm, J. (2012). The prevalence of mental health and pain symptoms in general population samples reporting nonmedical use of prescription opioids: A systematic review and meta-analysis. *The Journal of Pain, 13*(11), 1029–1044.

Fisher, W. H., Clark, R., Baxter, J., Barton, B., O'Connell, E., & Aweh, G. (2014). Co-occurring risk factors for arrest among persons with opioid abuse and dependence: Implications for developing interventions to limit criminal justice involvement. *Journal of Substance Abuse Treatment, 47*(3), 197–201.

Fischer, B., Murphy, Y., Kurdyak, P., & Goldner, E. M. (2016). Depression–A major but neglected consequence contributing to the health toll from prescription opioids? *Psychiatry Research, 243*, 331–334.

Florence, C., Luo, F., Xu, L., & Zhou, C. (2016). The economic burden of prescription opioid overdose, abuse and dependence in the United States, 2013. *Medical Care, 54*(10), 901.

Frank, R. G., & Pollack, H. A. (2017). Addressing the fentanyl threat to public health. *New England Journal of Medicine, 376*(7), 605–607.

Franklin, G. M. (2014). Opioids for chronic noncancer pain: A position paper of the American Academy of Neurology. *Neurology, 83*(14), 1277–1284.

Friedmann, P. D., Hoskinson, R., Jr., Gordon, M., Schwartz, R., Kinlock, T., Knight, K., et al. (2012). Medication-assisted treatment in criminal justice agencies affiliated with the criminal justice-drug abuse treatment studies (CJ-DATS): Availability, barriers, and intentions. *Substance Abuse, 33*(1), 9–18.

Fu, J. J., Zaller, N. D., Yokell, M. A., Bazazi, A. R., & Rich, J. D. (2013). Forced withdrawal from methadone maintenance therapy in criminal justice settings: A critical treatment barrier in the United States. *Journal of Substance Abuse Treatment, 44*(5), 502–505.

Galanie, S., Thodey, K., Trenchard, I. J., Interrante, M. F., & Smolke, C. D. (2015). Complete biosynthesis of opioids in yeast. *Science, 349*(6252), 1095–1100.

Garcia, C. A., Correa, G. C., Viver, A. D. H., Kinlock, T. W., Gordon, M. S., Avila, C. A., et al. (2007). Buprenorphine-naloxone treatment for pre-release opioid-dependent inmates in Puerto Rico. *Journal of Addiction Medicine, 1*(3), 126–132.

Gawande, A. A. (2017). It's time to adopt electronic prescriptions for opioids. *Annals of Surgery, 265*(4), 693–694.

Gomes, T., Juurlink, D. N., Antoniou, T., Mamdani, M. M., Paterson, J. M., & van den Brink, W. (2017). Gabapentin, opioids, and the risk of opioid-related death: A population-based nested case–control study. *PLoS Medicine, 14*(10), e1002396.

Grady, D., Berkowitz, S. A., & Katz, M. H. (2011). Opioids for chronic pain. *Archives of Internal Medicine, 171*(16), 1426–1427.

Grau, L. E., Dasgupta, N., Harvey, A. P., Irwin, K., Givens, A., Kinzly, M. L., & Heimer, R. (2007). Illicit use of opioids: Is OxyContin® a "gateway drug"? *The American Journal on Addictions, 16*(3), 166–173.

Gryczynski, J., Kinlock, T. W., Kelly, S. M., O'Grady, K. E., Gordon, M. S., & Schwartz, R. P. (2012). Opioid agonist maintenance for probationers: Patient-level predictors of treatment retention, drug use, and crime. *Substance Abuse, 33*(1), 30–39.

Hakansson, A., & Berglund, M. (2013). All-cause mortality in criminal justice clients with substance use problems—A prospective follow-up study. *Drug and Alcohol Dependence, 132*(3), 499–504.

Hakansson, A., Schlyter, F., & Berglund, M. (2008). Factors associated with history of non-fatal overdose among opioid users in the Swedish criminal justice system. *Drug and Alcohol Dependence, 94*(1–3), 48–55.

Hakansson, A., Schlyter, F., & Berglund, M. (2011). Associations between polysubstance use and psychiatric problems in a criminal justice population in Sweden. *Drug and Alcohol Dependence, 118*(1), 5–11.

Hall, W. D., & Farrell, M. P. (2011). Minimising the misuse of oxycodone and other pharmaceutical opioids in Australia. *The Medical Journal of Australia, 195*(5), 248–249.

Hansen, R. N., Oster, G., Edelsberg, J., Woody, G. E., & Sullivan, S. D. (2011). Economic costs of nonmedical use of prescription opioids. *The Clinical Journal of Pain, 27*(3), 194–202.

Hedrich, D., Alves, P., Farrell, M., Stöver, H., Møller, L., & Mayet, S. (2012). The effectiveness of opioid maintenance treatment in prison settings: A systematic review. *Addiction, 107*(3), 501–517.

Houry, D., & Baldwin, G. (2016). Announcing the CDC guideline for prescribing opioids for chronic pain. *Journal of Safety Research, 57*, 83–84.

Hser, Y. I., Evans, E., Grella, C., Ling, W., & Anglin, D. (2015). Long-term course of opioid addiction. *Harvard Review of Psychiatry, 23*(2), 76–89.

Jarlenski, M., Barry, C. L., Gollust, S., Graves, A. J., Kennedy-Hendricks, A., & Kozhimannil, K. (2017). Polysubstance use among US women of reproductive age who use opioids for nonmedical reasons. *American Journal of Public Health, 107*(8), 1308–1310.

Jensen-Dahm, C., Gasse, C., Astrup, A., Mortensen, P. B., & Waldemar, G. (2015). Frequent use of opioids in patients with dementia and nursing home residents: A study of the entire elderly population of Denmark. *Alzheimer's & Dementia, 11*(6), 691–699.

Jones, C. M., & McAninch, J. K. (2015). Emergency department visits and overdose deaths from combined use of opioids and benzodiazepines. *American Journal of Preventive Medicine, 49*(4), 493–501.

Katz, N. P., Birnbaum, H. G., & Castor, A. (2010). Volume of prescription opioids used nonmedically in the United States. *Journal of Pain & Palliative Care Pharmacotherapy, 24*(2), 141–144.

Katz, N., Dart, R. C., Bailey, E., Trudeau, J., Osgood, E., & Paillard, F. (2011). Tampering with prescription opioids: Nature and extent of the problem, health consequences, and solutions. *The American Journal of Drug and Alcohol Abuse, 37*(4), 205–217.

Kenan, K., Mack, K., & Paulozzi, L. (2012). Trends in prescriptions for oxycodone and other commonly used opioids in the United States, 2000–2010. *Open Medicine, 6*(2), e41.

Kharasch, E. D., & Brunt, L. M. (2016). Perioperative opioids and public health. *Anesthesiology: The Journal of the American Society of Anesthesiologists, 124*(4), 960–965.

Kolodny, A., Courtwright, D. T., Hwang, C. S., Kreiner, P., Eadie, J. L., Clark, T. W., & Alexander, G. C. (2015). The prescription opioid and heroin crisis: A public health approach to an epidemic of addiction. *Annual Review of Public Health, 36*, 559–574.

Koppen, L., Suda, K. J., Rowan, S., McGregor, J., & Evans, C. T. (2018). Dentists' prescribing of antibiotics and opioids to medicare part D beneficiaries: Medications of high impact to public health. *The Journal of the American Dental Association, 149*(8), 721–730.

Krawczyk, N., Picher, C. E., Feder, K. A., & Saloner, B. (2017). Only one in twenty justice-referred adults in specialty treatment for opioid use receive methadone or buprenorphine. *Health Affairs, 36*(12), 2046–2053.

Kuehn, B. M. (2010). Alarming nonfatal overdose rates found for opioids, sedatives, and tranquilizers. *JAMA, 303*(20), 2020–2021.

Larance, B., Degenhardt, L., Lintzeris, N., Winstock, A., & Mattick, R. (2011). Definitions related to the use of pharmaceutical opioids: Extramedical use, diversion, non-adherence and aberrant medication-related behaviours. *Drug and Alcohol Review, 30*(3), 236–245.

Larney, S. (2010). Does opioid substitution treatment in prisons reduce injecting-related HIV risk behaviours? A systematic review. *Addiction, 105*(2), 216–223.

Larney, S., Toson, B., Burns, L., & Dolan, K. (2012). Effect of prison-based opioid substitution treatment and post-release retention in treatment on risk of re-incarceration. *Addiction, 107*(2), 372–380.

Laxmaiah Manchikanti, M. D., Sairam Atluri, M. D., & Hans Hansen, M. D. (2014). Opioids in chronic noncancer pain: Have we reached a boiling point yet? *Pain Physician, 17*, E1–E10.

Lee, J. D., Friedmann, P. D., Boney, T. Y., Hoskinson, R. A., Jr., McDonald, R., Gordon, M., et al. (2015). Extended-release naltrexone to prevent relapse among opioid dependent, criminal justice system involved adults: Rationale and design of a randomized controlled effectiveness trial. *Contemporary Clinical Trials, 41*, 110–117.

Lee, J. D., Friedmann, P. D., Kinlock, T. W., Nunes, E. V., Boney, T. Y., Hoskinson, R. A., Jr., et al. (2016). Extended-release naltrexone to prevent opioid relapse in criminal justice offenders. *New England Journal of Medicine, 374*(13), 1232–1242.

Lee, J. D., McDonald, R., Grossman, E., McNeely, J., Laska, E., Rotrosen, J., & Gourevitch, M. N. (2015c). Opioid treatment at release from jail using extended-release naltrexone: A pilot proof-of-concept randomized effectiveness trial. *Addiction, 110*(6), 1008–1014.

Lembke, A. (2012). Why doctors prescribe opioids to known opioid abusers. *New England Journal of Medicine, 367*(17), 1580–1581.

Logie, D. E., & Harding, R. (2005). An evaluation of a morphine public health programme for cancer and AIDS pain relief in Sub-Saharan Africa. *BMC Public Health, 5*(1), 82.

Lucyk, S. N., & Nelson, L. S. (2017). Novel synthetic opioids: An opioid epidemic within an opioid epidemic. *Annals of Emergency Medicine, 69*(1), 91–93.

Manchikanti, L., & Singh, A. (2008). Therapeutic opioids: A ten-year perspective on the complexities and complications of the escalating use, abuse, and nonmedical use of opioids. *Pain Physician, 11*(2 Suppl), S63–S88.

Martin, C. E., Longinaker, N., & Terplan, M. (2015). Recent trends in treatment admissions for prescription opioid abuse during pregnancy. *Journal of Substance Abuse Treatment, 48*(1), 37–42.

Mateu-Gelabert, P., Guarino, H., Jessell, L., & Teper, A. (2015). Injection and sexual HIV/HCV risk behaviors associated with nonmedical use of prescription opioids among young adults in New York City. *Journal of Substance Abuse Treatment, 48*(1), 13–20.

McCabe, S. E., Boyd, C. J., Cranford, J. A., & Teter, C. J. (2009). Motives for nonmedical use of prescription opioids among high school seniors in the United States: Self-treatment and beyond. *Archives of Pediatrics & Adolescent Medicine, 163*(8), 739–744.

McCabe, S. E., Cranford, J. A., Boyd, C. J., & Teter, C. J. (2007). Motives, diversion and routes of administration associated with nonmedical use of prescription opioids. *Addictive Behaviors, 32*(3), 562–575.

McCabe, S. E., Teter, C. J., Boyd, C. J., Knight, J. R., & Wechsler, H. (2005). Nonmedical use of prescription opioids among US college students: Prevalence and correlates from a national survey. *Addictive Behaviors, 30*(4), 789–805.

McCabe, S. E., West, B. T., Teter, C. J., & Boyd, C. J. (2012). Co-ingestion of prescription opioids and other drugs among high school seniors: Results from a national study. *Drug and Alcohol Dependence, 126*(1–2), 65–70.

McCall Jones, C., Baldwin, G. T., & Compton, W. M. (2017). Recent increases in cocaine-related overdose deaths and the role of opioids. *American Journal of Public Health, 107*(3), 430–432.

McCarty, D., Perrin, N. A., Green, C. A., Polen, M. R., Leo, M. C., & Lynch, F. (2010). Methadone maintenance and the cost and utilization of health care among individuals dependent on opioids in a commercial health plan. *Drug and Alcohol Dependence, 111*(3), 235–240.

McLellan, A. T., & Turner, B. (2008). Prescription opioids, overdose deaths, and physician responsibility. *JAMA, 300*(22), 2672–2673.

Miech, R., Johnston, L., O'Malley, P. M., Keyes, K. M., & Heard, K. (2015). Prescription opioids in adolescence and future opioid misuse. *Pediatrics, 136*(5), e1169–e1177.

Mudumbai, S. C., Oliva, E. M., Lewis, E. T., Trafton, J., Posner, D., Mariano, E. R., et al. (2016). Time-to-cessation of postoperative opioids: A population-level analysis of the veterans affairs health care system. *Pain Medicine, 17*(9), 1732–1743.

Murphy, S. M., Polsky, D., Lee, J. D., Friedmann, P. D., Kinlock, T. W., Nunes, E. V., et al. (2017). Cost-effectiveness of extended release naltrexone to prevent relapse among criminal justice-involved individuals with a history of opioid use disorder. *Addiction, 112*(8), 1440–1450.

Nielsen, S., Lintzeris, N., Bruno, R., Campbell, G., Larance, B., Hall, W., et al. (2015). Benzodiazepine use among chronic pain patients prescribed opioids: Associations with pain, physical and mental health, and health service utilization. *Pain Medicine, 16*(2), 356–366.

O'Donnell, J. K., Gladden, R. M., & Seth, P. (2017). Trends in deaths involving heroin and synthetic opioids excluding methadone, and law enforcement drug product reports, by census region—United States, 2006–2015. *MMWR. Morbidity and Mortality Weekly Report, 66*(34), 897.

Oderda, G. M., Lake, J., Rüdell, K., Roland, C. L., & Masters, E. T. (2015). Economic burden of prescription opioid misuse and abuse: A systematic review. *Journal of Pain & Palliative Care Pharmacotherapy, 29*(4), 388–400.

Ogbu, U. C., Lotfipour, S., & Chakravarthy, B. (2015). Polysubstance abuse: Alcohol, opioids and benzodiazepines require coordinated engagement by society, patients, and physicians. *Western Journal of Emergency Medicine, 16*(1), 76–79.

Okie, S. (2010). A flood of opioids, a rising tide of deaths. *New England Journal of Medicine, 363*(21), 1981–1985.

Olsen, Y., & Sharfstein, J. M. (2014). Confronting the stigma of opioid use disorder—And its treatment. *JAMA, 311*(14), 1393–1394.

Patapis, N. S., & Nordstrom, B. R. (2006). Research on naltrexone in the criminal justice system. *Journal of Substance Abuse Treatment, 31*(2), 113–115.

Phillips, P. J., Smith, S. G., Kolpin, D. W., Zaugg, S. D., Buxton, H. T., Furlong, E. T., et al. (2010). Pharmaceutical formulation facilities as sources of opioids and other pharmaceuticals to wastewater treatment plant effluents. *Environmental Science & Technology, 44*(13), 4910–4916.

Pierce, M., Bird, S. M., Hickman, M., & Millar, T. (2015). National record linkage study of mortality for a large cohort of opioid users ascertained by drug treatment or criminal justice sources in England, 2005–2009. *Drug and Alcohol Dependence, 146*, 17–23.

Pollini, R. A., Banta-Green, C. J., Cuevas-Mota, J., Metzner, M., Teshale, E., & Garfein, R. S. (2011). Problematic use of prescription-type opioids prior to heroin use among young heroin injectors. *Substance Abuse and Rehabilitation, 2*, 173.

Popova, S., Patra, J., Mohapatra, S., Fischer, B., & Rehm, J. (2009). How many people in Canada use prescription opioids nonmedically in general and street drug using populations? *Canadian Journal of Public Health, 100*(2), 104–108.

Prekupec, M. P., Mansky, P. A., & Baumann, M. H. (2017). Misuse of novel synthetic opioids: A deadly new trend. *Journal of Addiction Medicine, 11*(4), 256.

Rajagopal, M. R., Joranson, D. E., & Gilson, A. M. (2001). Medical use, misues, and diversion of opioids in India. *The Lancet, 358*(9276), 139–143.

Reidenberg, M. M., & Willis, O. (2007). Prosecution of physicians for prescribing opioids to patients. *Clinical Pharmacology & Therapeutics, 81*(6), 903–906.

Reuben, D. B., Alvanzo, A. A., Ashikaga, T., Bogat, G. A., Callahan, C. M., Ruffing, V., & Steffens, D. C. (2015). National Institutes of health pathways to prevention workshop: The role of opioids in the treatment of chronic pain. *Annals of Internal Medicine, 162*(4), 295–300.

Robertson, A. G., Easter, M. M., Lin, H. J., Frisman, L. K., Swanson, J. W., & Swartz, M. S. (2018). Associations between pharmacotherapy for opioid dependence and clinical and criminal justice outcomes among adults with co-occurring serious mental illness. *Journal of Substance Abuse Treatment, 86*, 17–25.

Room, R., & Reuter, P. (2012). How well do international drug conventions protect public health? *The Lancet, 379*(9810), 84–91.

Savage, S. R., Joranson, D. E., Covington, E. C., Schnoll, S. H., Heit, H. A., & Gilson, A. M. (2003). Definitions related to the medical use of opioids: Evolution towards universal agreement. *Journal of Pain and Symptom Management, 26*(1), 655–667.

Schaub, M., Chtenguelov, V., Subata, E., Weiler, G., & Uchtenhagen, A. (2010). Feasibility of buprenorphine and methadone maintenance programmes among users of home made opioids in Ukraine. *International Journal of Drug Policy, 21*(3), 229–233.

Scherrer, J. F., Salas, J., Copeland, L. A., Stock, E. M., Schneider, F. D., Sullivan, M., et al. (2016). Increased risk of depression recurrence after initiation of prescription opioids in noncancer pain patients. *The Journal of Pain, 17*(4), 473–482.

Seal, K. H., Shi, Y., Cohen, G., Cohen, B. E., Maguen, S., Krebs, E. E., & Neylan, T. C. (2012). Association of mental health disorders with prescription opioids and high-risk opioid use in US veterans of Iraq and Afghanistan. *JAMA, 307*(9), 940–947.

Sepúlveda, C., Marlin, A., Yoshida, T., & Ullrich, A. (2002). Palliative care: The World Health Organization's global perspective. *Journal of Pain and Symptom Management, 24*(2), 91–96.

Seth, P., Scholl, L., Rudd, R. A., & Bacon, S. (2018). Overdose deaths involving opioids, cocaine, and psychostimulants—United States, 2015–2016. *Morbidity and Mortality Weekly Report, 67*(12), 349.

Shah, N. G., Lathrop, S. L., Reichard, R. R., & Landen, M. G. (2008). Unintentional drug overdose death trends in New Mexico, USA, 1990–2005: Combinations of heroin, cocaine, prescription opioids and alcohol. *Addiction, 103*(1), 126–136.

Sharma, A., Kelly, S. M., Mitchell, S. G., Gryczynski, J., O'Grady, K. E., & Schwartz, R. P. (2017). Update on barriers to pharmacotherapy for opioid use disorders. *Current Psychiatry Reports, 19*(6), 35.

Shei, A., Rice, J. B., Kirson, N. Y., Bodnar, K., Birnbaum, H. G., Holly, P., & Ben-Joseph, R. (2015). Sources of prescription opioids among diagnosed opioid abusers. *Current Medical Research and Opinion, 31*(4), 779–784.

Shield, K. D., Ialomiteanu, A., Fischer, B., Mann, R. E., & Rehm, J. (2011). Non-medical use of prescription opioids among Ontario adults: Data from the 2008/2009 CAMH monitor. *Canadian Journal of Public Health, 102*(5), 330–335.

Solomon, D. H., Rassen, J. A., Glynn, R. J., Garneau, K., Levin, R., Lee, J., & Schneeweiss, S. (2010). The comparative safety of opioids for nonmalignant pain in older adults. *Archives of Internal Medicine, 170*(22), 1979–1986.

Springer, S. A., Qiu, J., Saber-Tehrani, A. S., & Altice, F. L. (2012). Retention on buprenorphine is associated with high levels of maximal viral suppression among HIV-infected opioid dependent released prisoners. *PLoS One, 7*(5), e38335.

Stanos, S. P., Bruckenthal, P., & Barkin, R. L. (2012, July). Strategies to reduce the tampering and subsequent abuse of long-acting opioids: Potential risks and benefits of formulations with physical or pharmacologic deterrents to tampering. In *Mayo Clinic Proceedings* (Vol. 87, No. 7, pp. 683–694). Elsevier.

Stjernswärd, J., Foley, K. M., & Ferris, F. D. (2007). The public health strategy for palliative care. *Journal of Pain and Symptom Management, 33*(5), 486–493.

Stover, M. W., & Davis, J. M. (2015, November). Opioids in pregnancy and neonatal abstinence syndrome. In *Seminars in Perinatology* (Vol. 39, No. 7, pp. 561–565). WB Saunders.

Strassels, S. (2009). Economic burden of prescription opioid misuse and abuse. *Journal of Managed Care Pharmacy, 15*(7), 556–562.

Subramaniam, G. A., & Stitzer, M. A. (2009). Clinical characteristics of treatment-seeking prescription opioid vs. heroin-using adolescents with opioid use disorder. *Drug and Alcohol Dependence, 101*(1–2), 13–19.

Sun, E. C., Dixit, A., Humphreys, K., Darnall, B. D., Baker, L. C., & Mackey, S. (2017). Association between concurrent use of prescription opioids and benzodiazepines and overdose: Retrospective analysis. *BMJ, 356*, j760.

The, M. T. C., Swetz, A., of Correction, M. D, Kinlock, T. W., Battjes, R. J., & Schwartz, R. P. (2002). A novel opioid maintenance program for prisoners: Preliminary findings. *Journal of Substance Abuse Treatment, 22*(3), 141–147.

Van Zee, A. (2009). The promotion and marketing of oxycontin: Commercial triumph, public health tragedy. *American Journal of Public Health, 99*(2), 221–227.

Von Korff, M. (2013a). Opioids for chronic musculoskeletal pain: Putting patient safety first. *Pain, 154*(12), 2583.

Von Korff, M. R. (2013b). Long-term use of opioids for complex chronic pain. *Best Practice & Research Clinical Rheumatology, 27*(5), 663–672.

Wagner, K. D., Liu, L., Davidson, P. J., Cuevas-Mota, J., Armenta, R. F., & Garfein, R. S. (2015). Association between non-fatal opioid overdose and encounters with healthcare and criminal justice systems: Identifying opportunities for intervention. *Drug and Alcohol Dependence, 153*, 215–220.

Wall, R., Rehm, J., Fischer, B., Gliksman, L., Stewart, J., Medved, W., & Blake, J. (2000). Social costs of untreated opioid dependence. *Journal of Urban Health, 77*(4), 688–722.

Wang, K. H., Becker, W. C., & Fiellin, D. A. (2013). Prevalence and correlates for nonmedical use of prescription opioids among urban and rural residents. *Drug and Alcohol Dependence, 127*(1–3), 156–162.

Winkelman, T. N., Chang, V. W., & Binswanger, I. A. (2018). Health, polysubstance use, and criminal justice involvement among adults with varying levels of opioid use. *JAMA Network Open, 1*(3), e180558.

Wu, L. T., Blazer, D. G., Li, T. K., & Woody, G. E. (2011). Treatment use and barriers among adolescents with prescription opioid use disorders. *Addictive Behaviors, 36*(12), 1233–1239.

Wunsch, H., Wijeysundera, D. N., Passarella, M. A., & Neuman, M. D. (2016). Opioids prescribed after low-risk surgical procedures in the United States, 2004-2012. *JAMA, 315*(15), 1654–1657.

Wunsch, M. J., Cropsey, K. L., Campbell, E. D., & Knisely, J. S. (2008). OxyContin use and misuse in three populations: Substance abuse patients, pain patients, and criminal justice participants. *Journal of Opioid Management, 4*(2), 73–79.

Yazdy, M. M., Mitchell, A. A., Tinker, S. C., Parker, S. E., & Werler, M. M. (2013). Periconceptional use of opioids and the risk of neural tube defects. *Obstetrics and Ggynecology, 122*(4), 838.

Young, A. M., Havens, J. R., & Leukefeld, C. G. (2010). Route of administration for illicit prescription opioids: A comparison of rural and urban drug users. *Harm Reduction Journal, 7*(1), 24.

Young, A., McCabe, S. E., Cranford, J. A., Ross-Durow, P., & Boyd, C. J. (2012). Nonmedical use of prescription opioids among adolescents: Subtypes based on motivation for use. *Journal of Addictive Diseases, 31*(4), 332–341.

Zedler, B., Xie, L., Wang, L., Joyce, A., Vick, C., Kariburyo, F., et al. (2014). Risk factors for serious prescription opioid-related toxicity or overdose among veterans health administration patients. *Pain Medicine, 15*(11), 1911–1929.

Index

W. G. Jennings et al., *Opioid Prescribing Rates and Criminal Justice and Health Outcomes*, SpringerBriefs in Criminology,
https://doi.org/10.1007/978-3-030-40764-3